CANCER ETIOLOGY, DIAGNOSIS AND TREATMENTS

MESOTHELIOMA

RISK FACTORS, TREATMENT AND PROGNOSIS

CANCER ETIOLOGY, DIAGNOSIS AND TREATMENTS

Additional books and e-books in this series can be found on Nova's website under the Series tab.

CANCER ETIOLOGY, DIAGNOSIS AND TREATMENTS

MESOTHELIOMA

RISK FACTORS, TREATMENT AND PROGNOSIS

ALBERT K. MARTIN
EDITOR

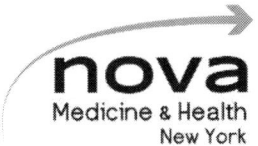

Copyright © 2021 by Nova Science Publishers, Inc.
https://doi.org/10.52305/FRKL1404

All rights reserved. No part of this book may be reproduced, stored in a retrieval system or transmitted in any form or by any means: electronic, electrostatic, magnetic, tape, mechanical photocopying, recording or otherwise without the written permission of the Publisher.

We have partnered with Copyright Clearance Center to make it easy for you to obtain permissions to reuse content from this publication. Simply navigate to this publication's page on Nova's website and locate the "Get Permission" button below the title description. This button is linked directly to the title's permission page on copyright.com. Alternatively, you can visit copyright.com and search by title, ISBN, or ISSN.

For further questions about using the service on copyright.com, please contact:
Copyright Clearance Center
Phone: +1-(978) 750-8400   Fax: +1-(978) 750-4470   E-mail: info@copyright.com.

NOTICE TO THE READER

The Publisher has taken reasonable care in the preparation of this book, but makes no expressed or implied warranty of any kind and assumes no responsibility for any errors or omissions. No liability is assumed for incidental or consequential damages in connection with or arising out of information contained in this book. The Publisher shall not be liable for any special, consequential, or exemplary damages resulting, in whole or in part, from the readers' use of, or reliance upon, this material. Any parts of this book based on government reports are so indicated and copyright is claimed for those parts to the extent applicable to compilations of such works.

Independent verification should be sought for any data, advice or recommendations contained in this book. In addition, no responsibility is assumed by the Publisher for any injury and/or damage to persons or property arising from any methods, products, instructions, ideas or otherwise contained in this publication.

This publication is designed to provide accurate and authoritative information with regard to the subject matter covered herein. It is sold with the clear understanding that the Publisher is not engaged in rendering legal or any other professional services. If legal or any other expert assistance is required, the services of a competent person should be sought. FROM A DECLARATION OF PARTICIPANTS JOINTLY ADOPTED BY A COMMITTEE OF THE AMERICAN BAR ASSOCIATION AND A COMMITTEE OF PUBLISHERS.

Additional color graphics may be available in the e-book version of this book.

Library of Congress Cataloging-in-Publication Data

ISBN: 978-1-68507-075-5

Published by Nova Science Publishers, Inc. † New York

Contents

Preface		vii
Chapter 1	Mesothelioma: The Advent of Immunotherapy *Luca Cantini, Federica Pecci, Edoardo Lenci, Valeria Cognigni and Rossana Berardi*	1
Chapter 2	Malignant Mesothelioma *Anwar M. Alesawi, Faisal S. Mandourah and Hasan M. Alesawi*	51
Chapter 3	Inflammatory and Immunological Aspects in the Surgical Management of Malignant Pleural Mesothelioma *Riccardo Tajè, Federico Tacconi, Roberto Fiorito, Alessandro Tamburrini and Vincenzo Ambrogi*	87
Chapter 4	New Developments in Mesothelioma Markers *Gregorio Bonsignore, Simona Martinotti, Federica Grosso and Elia Ranzato*	115
Chapter 5	Surgical Approaches to Pleural Tumours *Elena Prisciandaro, Luca Bertolaccini, Lara Girelli and Lorenzo Spaggiari*	141
Index		159

Preface

Mesothelioma is a type of cancer in which tumors form in the tissue that lines the lungs, heart, stomach, and other organs. While mesothelioma is relatively rare, it represents a serious health crisis as the disease is aggressive and often fatal. This book includes five chapters that detail the treatment and prognosis of the disease as well as the factors that put a person at risk for developing mesothelioma. Chapter one describes the most promising emerging immunotherapy combinations for the treatment of malignant pleural mesothelioma, discussing the biological rational underlying their development as well as the issues surrounding their clinical development. Chapter two provides an overview of malignant mesothelioma, describing the history of its diagnosis and treatment as well as the role that asbestos exposure and other factors play in its development. Chapter three revises the role of the main inflammatory and immunological markers as prognostic indicators in malignant pleural mesothelioma and discusses the surgical effects on immune response against cancer. Chapter four explores the main cancer markers utilized for mesothelioma diagnosis as well as the new developments in the field. Lastly, Chapter five examines the various surgical options available for removing pleural tumors.

Chapter 1 - Malignant pleural mesothelioma (MPM) is a rare but aggressive and treatment resistant neoplasm with low survival rates. The limited benefit of available treatments (platinum-based chemotherapy) together with an exponential growth in the appreciation of mesothelioma pathobiology, prompted the investigation of new therapeutic strategies both in the early stage of the disease and in the advanced setting. Considering the important role which the immune system exerts in the pathogenesis of MPM, expectations are now high that immunotherapy and in particular immune check-point inhibitors (ICIs) will have a leading role in the next few years. However, promising results with ICI monotherapy from phase II studies in MPM were often not replicated in larger, randomized, phase III trials. The alternating results of ICI monotherapy might be due to the lack of biomarkers able to identify patients more likely to benefit from ICI treatment, as well as to the immunogenic characteristics of MPM. Results of the phase III Checkmate743 randomized trial, which firstly demonstrated the superiority of ICI combination (nivolumab plus ipilimumab) over chemotherapy in first-line treatment for unresectable MPM patients, showed that combining immunotherapies might be a successful strategy to overcome resistance. In this chapter, the authors describe the most promising emerging immunotherapy combinations for the treatment of MPM, discussing the biological rationale underlying their development as well as the issues surrounding their clinical development.

Chapter 2 - Malignant Mesothelioma (MM) is an insidious neoplasm arising from mesothelial surfaces i.e., pleura (65%-70%), peritoneum (30%), tunica vaginalis testis, and pericardium (1%-2%). It is a rare but rapidly fatal and aggressive tumor with limited knowledge of its natural history. The earliest mention of a possible tumor of the chest wall (the pleura) was made in 1767 by Joseph Lieutaud, while Peritoneal mesothelioma was first described in 1908 by Miller and Wynn. The incidence is approximately 2500 per year in the United States. Comparing to lung cancer, incidence is more than 160,000 new cases per year. Asbestos exposure plays a critical role in malignant pleural mesothelioma in the United States. There are several risk factors that linked to development of malignant mesothelioma like ionizing radiation, genetic susceptibility, exposure to particular viruses like simian virus 40, but still occupational and environmental asbestos exposure remains a major causative factor. Treatment of malignant mesothelioma range from surgery to radiation and chemotherapy, but preventive measures like taking the appropriate precautions if you are exposed to asbestos at work is a major part of management.

Chapter 3 - Malignant Pleural Mesothelioma is an aggressive cancer. Extrapleural pneumonectomy and extended pleurectomy/decortication are the two intentionally-radical surgical strategies, burdened with different complication rates. Both procedures fail to obtain true microscopic radical resection, achieving similar results in terms of disease-free and overall survivals. Therefore, decision over the best surgical approach remains equivocal. With the increasing knowledge regarding the influence of inflammation and immunity in carcinogenesis processes, several inflammatory markers gained prognostic values and currently affect therapeutic decisions and treatment strategies. Growing evidence supports the prognostic role of inflammatory markers such as neutrophils-to-lymphocytes ratio, platelets-to-lymphocytes ratio, albumin and C reactive protein in malignant pleural mesothelioma. Comprehensive and established prognostic scores including inflammatory markers may help surgeons to stratify patients pre-operatively. Nonetheless, the effects of surgery on cancer immunity are debatable. Post-operative systemic inflammation may indeed hinder the immune system leading to immuno-tolerance, but on the contrary, surgical debulking may expose immunogenic epitope re-activating host defences against cancerous cells. A better knowledge and a more thorough understanding of this immunological balance could empower surgery with new significances, as surgery could both extirpate gross masses and function as an immunotherapy or radiotherapy booster in a multimodal treatment. In this report the authors revise the role of the main inflammatory and immunological markers as prognostic indicators in malignant pleural mesothelioma. The authors also discuss the surgical effects on immune response against cancer.

Chapter 4 - Malignant mesothelioma is a rare cancer arising from serosal surface of the body. Its incidence is strictly related to asbestos exposure, that confers a long-term risk of developing this cancer. So, due to poor therapy options and long latency time for exposure, there is an urgent need to explore new markers for mesothelioma diagnosis and treatment follow-up. In this chapter, the authors will explore the main cancer markers utilized for mesothelioma diagnosis as well as the new developments in the field.

Chapter 5 - The pleurae are serous membranes encasing the lungs and may develop benign and malignant neoplasms. Primary pleural tumours may arise in the visceral pleura, the parietal pleura, or both. Benign tumours are usually confined to the pleura, rarely causing infiltration of the surrounding tissues or distant metastases and has a surgical treatment. The most common one is malignant pleural mesothelioma (MPM). Mesothelioma is a malignant neoplasm that originates from the mesothelia, the lining sheets of the serous cavities: pleura, pericardium, peritoneum and, in men, the tunica vaginalis of the testicles. In more than 90% of cases, mesothelioma has a pleural localisation (MPM). The current standard-of-care treatment of MPM is generally accepted as systemic therapy alone. Surgery could be part of a multimodal treatment plan since it is the only modality that could render a patient without the disease. Selecting patients fit for surgery, determining the optimal operation, and the additional treatments have not yet been established due to the extreme variability of cancer itself related to the variability of the surgical techniques. The complete macroscopic resection is the objective of surgical treatment. Surgery (open or VATS pleural biopsies) could help achieve an MPM correct diagnosis or palliate (VATS pleurectomy, VATS talc pleurodesis, indwelling pleural drainage placement) symptoms caused by malignant pleural effusions. Every time aggressive surgery is scheduled, it aims to remove all visible disease, increasing survival by decreasing the intrathoracic tumour burden to microscopic levels. Ideally, all MPM patients should be operated on by Thoracic Surgeons with recognised broad experience in MPM management, regularly related to Radiation and Medical Oncology involved in MPM clinical trials. Even though there is a brand new, improved MPM staging system, the results of surgery for MPM are strongly influenced by other prognosticators not taken by the current staging system (such as subtype of histology). Consequently, at this time it is not possible to determine a common denominator that permits laborious evaluation between surgical series and ultimate establishing which surgical approach and adjuvants are advantageous and in which sequences/circumstances used or combined.

In: Mesothelioma
Editor: Albert K. Martin

ISBN: 978-1-68507-075-5
© 2021 Nova Science Publishers, Inc.

Chapter 1

MESOTHELIOMA: THE ADVENT OF IMMUNOTHERAPY

Luca Cantini[*]*, MD, Federica Pecci, MD, Edoardo Lenci, MD, Valeria Cognigni, MD* **and** *Rossana Berardi, MD*
Clinical Oncology, Università Politecnica Delle Marche,
AOU Ospedali Riuniti Ancona, Ancona, Italy

ABSTRACT

Malignant pleural mesothelioma (MPM) is a rare but aggressive and treatment resistant neoplasm with low survival rates. The limited benefit of available treatments (platinum-based chemotherapy) together with an exponential growth in the appreciation of mesothelioma pathobiology, prompted the investigation of new therapeutic strategies both in the early stage of the disease and in the advanced setting.

---

[*] Corresponding Author's E-mail: lucacantini.med@gmail.com.

Considering the important role which the immune system exerts in the pathogenesis of MPM, expectations are now high that immunotherapy and in particular immune check-point inhibitors (ICIs) will have a leading role in the next few years. However, promising results with ICI monotherapy from phase II studies in MPM were often not replicated in larger, randomized, phase III trials. The alternating results of ICI monotherapy might be due to the lack of biomarkers able to identify patients more likely to benefit from ICI treatment, as well as to the immunogenic characteristics of MPM.

Results of the phase III Checkmate743 randomized trial, which firstly demonstrated the superiority of ICI combination (nivolumab plus ipilimumab) over chemotherapy in first-line treatment for unresectable MPM patients, showed that combining immunotherapies might be a successful strategy to overcome resistance. In this chapter, we describe the most promising emerging immunotherapy combinations for the treatment of MPM, discussing the biological rationale underlying their development as well as the issues surrounding their clinical development.

Keywords: malignant pleural mesothelioma, immunotherapy, immune check-point inhibitors

INTRODUCTION

Malignant pleural mesothelioma (MPM) is an uncommon and orphan thoracic malignancy, whose incidence ranges between 10 cases per million to 29 cases per million depending on the country. Because the onset symptoms are not specific, MPM patients are often detected at a late stage and median survival time from first signs of illness to death remains around 12 months[1]. Even in patients in whom the disease is detected in an early phase, survival is not prolonged, and early diagnosis does not always lead to an increase in survival with the current treatment options. Contrary to other cancers, MPM has a peculiar pathogenesis, as a direct causal

---

[1] Robinson, Musk, and Lake, "Malignant Mesothelioma."

relationship between exposure to airborne asbestos particles and the development of MPM can be established in almost 90% of the cases[2].

The persistence of asbestos fibers in the pleural cavity results in chronic inflammation and eventually in oncogenic transformation of mesothelial cells[3]. In the last two decades, a better appreciation of mesothelioma biology has revealed the key role of the immune system in development and progression of MPM. This fact, along with the gradual introduction of immunotherapy in cancer treatment, has encouraged the investigation of agents able to harness the potency and the specificity of the immune system also in MPM patients.

Results from a prespecified interim analysis of a phase III randomized trial (Checkmate743) comparing the combination of two immune checkpoint inhibitors (ICIs) nivolumab and ipilimumab vs standard platinum-based chemotherapy in treatment-naive unresectable MPM recently corroborated the potential of immunotherapy in the first-line setting and led to the recent approval by the Food and Drug Administration (FDA) for this combination[4]. This breakthrough study made the pair with the CONFIRM trial which investigated the role of nivolumab in the salvage setting and reported a survival benefit over placebo[5]. It is now then clear that ICIs (and possibly other immunotherapies) will be central in future therapeutic choices for MPM patients. However, it is unlikely that all patients will similarly benefit from it and alternative strategies are needed to develop more tailored approaches and counteract treatment resistance.

Next chapters summarize the current status of knowledge in mesothelioma immune-biology, as well as past, present, and future studies in the field of immunotherapy for MPM.

---

[2] JC, CA, and P, "Diffuse Pleural Mesothelioma and Asbestos Exposure in the North Western Cape Province."
[3] M and H, "Molecular Pathways: Targeting Mechanisms of Asbestos and Erionite Carcinogenesis in Mesothelioma."
[4] P et al., "First-Line Nivolumab plus Ipilimumab in Unresectable Malignant Pleural Mesothelioma (CheckMate 743): A Multicentre, Randomised, Open-Label, Phase 3 Trial."
[5] Fennell et al., "PS01.11 Nivolumab Versus Placebo in Relapsed Malignant Mesothelioma: The CONFIRM Phase 3 Trial."

Rationale: Immune Cells Orchestra inside Mesothelioma Tumor Microenvironment

The origin of MPM is strictly linked to inflammatory response. In fact, asbestos exposure is considered the main risk factor for developing this rare type of cancer and inflammatory cells and their secretome hold a key role both in the initiation and progression of MPM (Figure 1).

Inhaled asbestos fibers migrate to pleural space and interact with mesothelial cells and immune cells, establishing a process of chronic inflammation with a latency of up to 30-40 years from exposure to MPM diagnosis[6]. Inside pleural space, asbestos fibers are phagocytized by macrophages, and because these cells are unable to totally digest them, this fact leads to the production of reactive oxygen species (ROS). Moreover, asbestos has direct effect on mesothelial cells leading to DNA damage and strand breaks, damage enhanced at the same time by ROS derived from both asbestos fibers and macrophages[7]. A storm of inflammatory cytokines and growth factors, released by asbestos-exposed mesothelial cells and macrophages, spreads locally and, attracting and activating a wide spectrum of immune and stromal cells, leads to MPM carcinogenesis, tumor progression and the shaping of a unique tumor microenvironment (TME)[8].

Several studies investigated the effects of asbestos fibers on immune cells, observing that continued exposure of T lymphocytes to asbestos fibers impaired anti-tumor activity of both CD8+ and CD4+ T cells[9]. Kumagai-Takei N. and colleagues demonstrated that exposure to asbestos suppresses the differentiation of cytotoxic T lymphocytes, in association with a lower production of interferon-gamma (IFN-gamma) and tumor

---

[6] Y, "Molecular Pathogenesis of Malignant Mesothelioma."
[7] TA et al., "Novel Insights into Mesothelioma Biology and Implications for Therapy."
[8] H, JR, and M, "Mesothelioma Epidemiology, Carcinogenesis, and Pathogenesis."
[9] N et al., "The Effects of Asbestos Fibers on Human T Cells."

necrosis factor-alpha (TNF-alpha), thus impairing their anti-tumor activity[10].

Therefore, the deep link between MPM and the immune system, rooted in the origin of MPM itself, suggests a possible role of immunotherapy in the fight of this rare and lethal neoplasm.

The MPM TME tends to acquire an immunosuppressive and anergic profile, leading to the growth of cancer cells that are more resistant to both chemotherapy and immunological treatments[11]. A key role is detained by soluble factors, such as cytokines and chemokines, that orchestrate the immune cells influx and differentiation inside TME[12]. Chéné AL et al.[13] demonstrated that C-C motif chemokine ligand 2 (CCL2) inflammatory chemokine and macrophage colony-stimulating factor (M-CSF) promote monocyte recruitment and differentiation of macrophages toward a pro-tumorigenic and immunosuppressive phenotype (M2 macrophages) in pleural mesothelioma. Another work by Khanna S et al. showed that tumor-derived granulocyte-macrophage colony-stimulating factor (GM-CSF) is able to boost the release of ROS from granulocytes, resulting in T-cell suppression inside TME.

Macrophages play a key role both in the development, progression and dismal prognosis of MPM. Tumor associated macrophages (TAMs) are numerous in MPM tissue, with about 25-40% of total immune infiltrates[14] and boost the immunosuppressive phenotype of TME[15].

The phenotypes of TAMs are dynamic and rely on the local microenvironment. TAMs are characterized by special receptor tyrosine kinases, such as Tyro3, Axl, and MerTK, important for interacting with

---

[10] N et al., "Effect of Asbestos Exposure on Differentiation of Cytotoxic T Lymphocytes in Mixed Lymphocyte Reaction of Human Peripheral Blood Mononuclear Cells."
[11] IC et al., "Potential Diagnostic and Prognostic Role of Microenvironment in Malignant Pleural Mesothelioma."
[12] GJ, N, and JEJ, "The Immune Microenvironment in Mesothelioma: Mechanisms of Resistance to Immunotherapy."
[13] AL et al., "Pleural Effusions from Patients with Mesothelioma Induce Recruitment of Monocytes and Their Differentiation into M2 Macrophages."
[14] J et al., "Heterogeneity in Immune Cell Content in Malignant Pleural Mesothelioma."
[15] A et al., "Phenotypic and Functional Analysis of Malignant Mesothelioma Tumor-Infiltrating Lymphocytes."

tumor cells and also macrophage polarization and they share several properties with M2 macrophages[16].

A recent work by Horio D et al.[17] demonstrated that TAMs are able to secrete interleukin-1beta (IL-1β) in the MPM microenvironment, leading to higher expression of cancer stem cell marker CD26 on mesothelioma cells, making them more resistant to chemotherapy treatments[18]. Moreover, they promote the infiltration of Regulatory T cells (Tregs) inside TME. Numbers of stromal macrophages were positively correlated to the number of stromal Tregs[19,20]; in fact, it has been proved that TAMs recruit Tregs through CCL22[21], which further suppress the antitumor activity of T-cells.

Colony-Stimulating Factor 1 (CSF1)/Colony-Stimulating Factor Receptor (CSF1R) signaling also detains a key role in the differentiation of monocytes into specific TAM phenotypes[22] and alters CD8$^+$ T cell cytotoxicity[23]. A preclinical study demonstrated how CSF1/CSF1R axis blockade inhibits tumor progression, macrophage tumor infiltration, induces macrophage polarization toward M1 phenotype and activates tumor dendritic cells. Therefore, CSF1R inhibition, combined with programmed death ligand 1 (PD-L1) inhibitors, might be a promising immunotherapeutic against MPM[24].

The prognostic significance of macrophages is still under investigation among MPM histotypes. Cornelissen R and colleagues showed that the CD163/CD68 ratio (CD68+ positive cells representing all macrophages phenotypes and CD163+ representing M2 phenotype) rather than the total

---

[16] J et al., "Tumor-Associated Macrophages: Recent Insights and Therapies."
[17] D et al., "Tumor-Associated Macrophage-Derived Inflammatory Cytokine Enhances Malignant Potential of Malignant Pleural Mesothelioma."
[18] S, A, and A, "CD26 a Cancer Stem Cell Marker and Therapeutic Target."
[19] J et al., "Heterogeneity in Immune Cell Content in Malignant Pleural Mesothelioma."
[20] E et al., "Prognostic and Predictive Aspects of the Tumor Immune Microenvironment and Immune Checkpoints in Malignant Pleural Mesothelioma."
[21] TJ et al., "Specific Recruitment of Regulatory T Cells in Ovarian Carcinoma Fosters Immune Privilege and Predicts Reduced Survival."
[22] T et al., "Involvement of the M-CSF/IL-34/CSF-1R Pathway in Malignant Pleural Mesothelioma."
[23] Y et al., "CSF1/CSF1R Blockade Reprograms Tumor-Infiltrating Macrophages and Improves Response to T-Cell Checkpoint Immunotherapy in Pancreatic Cancer Models."
[24] SF et al., "CSF1/CSF1R Axis Blockade Limits Mesothelioma and Enhances Efficiency of Anti-PDL1 Immunotherapy."

number of macrophages in MPM tumor tissue, correlates with overall survival (OS) in epithelioid MPM patients[25]. Another work by Burt et al. showed that the absolute number of CD68+ macrophages was linked with bad prognosis in non-epithelioid MPM[26].

Interestingly, a recent study by Pezzuto F et al. recognized a subgroup of MPM characterized by immunohistochemical p14/ARF expression, a tumor suppressor protein encoded by CDKN2A gene, one of the most frequently reported genomic alteration in MPM. They analyzed the immune TME and found that p14/ARF-negative tumors seem to detain a more immunosuppressive immune microenvironment, associated with low PD-L1 and high $CD163^+$ macrophages percentage, improving our knowledge about the potential link between molecular alterations and immune cells infiltration inside TME[27].

Myeloid-derived suppressor cells (MDSCs) have a key role in shaping of MPM TME and consist both in polymorphonuclear (PMN-MDSC) or monocytic (M-MDSC)[28]. They act as suppressive anti-tumor immune cells inhibiting T-cell activity by ROS production; moreover PD-L1 expression on their surface is associated with lower concentration of T-cells in the TME[29]. MDSCs promote tumor progression by stimulating transforming growth factor-beta (TGF-β), epidermal growth factor (EGF), and hepatocyte growth factor (HGF) signaling pathways, leading to epithelial–mesenchymal transition (EMT) of cancer cells, angiogenesis[30,31], inhibiting the anti-tumor activity of natural killer (NK) cells, and recruiting other

---

[25] R et al., "Ratio of Intratumoral Macrophage Phenotypes Is a Prognostic Factor in Epithelioid Malignant Pleural Mesothelioma."
[26] F et al., "Pathological Characterization of Tumor Immune Microenvironment (TIME) in Malignant Pleural Mesothelioma."
[27] F et al., "P14/ARF-Positive Malignant Pleural Mesothelioma: A Phenotype with Distinct Immune Microenvironment."
[28] ED and SI, "Granulocytic Myeloid-Derived Suppressor Cells as Negative Regulators of Anticancer Immunity."
[29] ED and SI.
[30] B et al., "Mesenchymal Transition and Dissemination of Cancer Cells Is Driven by Myeloid-Derived Suppressor Cells Infiltrating the Primary Tumor."
[31] A et al., "Myeloid Derived Suppressor Cells Interactions with Natural Killer Cells and Pro-Angiogenic Activities: Roles in Tumor Progression."

immunosuppressive cells[32]. In co-culture with CD8$^+$ T-cells from the same MPM tissue, both Gr-MDSCs and Mo-MDSCs reduced CD8$^+$ T-cell IFN-production and proliferation, leading them to a state of energy. Moreover, due to the higher production of ROS, Nitric oxide (NO) and kynurenine, MDSCs boost the immunosuppressive effect on T-cells[33].

This work also showed that MDSCs concentration inside TME detains a prognostic value: high intratumoral Treg, granulocytic myeloid-derived suppressor cells (Gr-MDSCs) and monocytic myeloid-derived suppressor cells (Mo-MDSCs) significantly correlated with shorter progression free survival (PFS) and OS in a cohort of MPMs; on the other hand, MDSCs concentration in pleural fluid did not show any significant correlation with patient survival.

Dendritic cells (DCs) are essential for antigen presentation to T cells and, therefore, for an appropriate anti-tumor immune response. It has been shown that DCs inside MPM TME are dysfunctional, leading to an impaired antigen presentation and subsequent cytotoxic T-cell action.

Gardner JK and colleagues showed how mesothelioma tumor cells modulate DCs activity. They observed that immature human monocyte-derived DCs (MoDCs) exposed to mesothelioma tumor cells and their secreted factors were characterized by an higher lipid content compared to control DCs and lipid accumulation was associated with reduced antigen processing ability and production of the tolerogenic cytokine, such as IL-10, impairing the ability of DCs to generate effective anti-mesothelioma T cell response[34].

Boosting the antigen-processing ability and exploiting immunostimulatory capacities of DCs are under investigation in several clinical trials to improve immune response against mesothelioma cells. Interestingly, a deep link between intracellular pathways involved also in metabolic

---

[32] D and DI, "Myeloid-Derived Suppressor Cells in the Tumor Microenvironment: Expect the Unexpected."
[33] IC et al., "Potential Diagnostic and Prognostic Role of Microenvironment in Malignant Pleural Mesothelioma."
[34] JK et al., "Mesothelioma Tumor Cells Modulate Dendritic Cell Lipid Content, Phenotype and Function."

functions and immune cells activity has been shown in pre-clinical models. Moreover, drugs implied in metabolic regulation seem to be also involved in immunogenicity regulation. Statins are able to inhibit the mevalonate (MVA) pathway involved in the production of cholesterol, and also interfere with prenylation, a posttranslational modification, of small GTPases proteins, altering their internal cell membrane anchorage and, therefore, arresting endocytic vesicles trafficking[35]. Therefore, statins might prolong antigen retention on cell membranes and boost antigen presentation to T cells, thus suggesting a potential synergic effect with PD-1 inhibitors, as shown in a retrospective study of patients affected by MPM and treated with immune checkpoints inhibitors[36]. Further studies are needed to deeply understand the link between intracellular metabolic pathways and immune cells activity in MPM, paving the way to the development of forefront drugs combinations.

Lymphocytes represent another heterogenous subpopulation of immune cells that contribute to tumor suppression or tumor progression inside TME.

An interesting work by Klampatsa A et al. carried out a phenotypic and functional analysis of tumor-infiltrating lymphocytes (TILs) in MPM TME. They collected fresh tumor and blood from 22 MPM patients and analyzed single cell suspensions by flow cytometry. They found a high percentage of exhausted T-cells: among CD8+ T cells, programmed death 1 (PD-1) was expressed in about ~50%, TIM-3 ~ in about 20%. They also detected the expression of other inhibitory receptors such as T cell immunoreceptor with Ig and ITIM domains protein (TIGIT), CD39 and Cytotoxic T-Lymphocyte Antigen 4 (CTLA4), expressed by ~60%, ~20% and ~25% of CD8+ T cells respectively.

Compared to T cells from healthy lung tissue, cytotoxic T cells in MPM express more TIGIT and TIM-3 compared to T cells from healthy

---

[35] Y et al., "The Mevalonate Pathway Is a Druggable Target for Vaccine Adjuvant Discovery."
[36] L et al., "High-Intensity Statins Are Associated with Improved Clinical Activity of PD-1 Inhibitors in Malignant Pleural Mesothelioma and Advanced Non-Small Cell Lung Cancer Patients."

lung tissue and had a minor ability to produce IFN-gamma upon stimulation, suggesting a hypofunctional state of MPM TILs.

Moreover, around 12.8% of CD4+ T cells in MPM tissues were positive for FoxP3 compared to 2.2% from healthy lung tissue, suggesting a more immunosuppressive microenvironment[37].

Both TILs quantitative infiltration and phenotype seem to also detain a prognostic value.

In a cohort of 308 MPM samples, high TILs (CD4+ and CD8+ T cells) infiltration correlated with non-epithelioid histology, greater expression of PD-L1 and PD-L2 and worse prognosis[38].

Pasello G et al. provided a deep description of immune cell heterogeneity inside TME and they showed that sarcomatoid and biphasic MPM samples were characterized by higher $CD8^+$ T cells, while epithelioid showed higher peritumoral $CD4^+$ T and $CD20^+$ B lymphocytes. They generated a pathological score composed by $CD8^+$ T lymphocytes, necrosis, mitosis, and proliferation index and found that patients with an high combined score detained an OS of 11.3 months compared with an OS of 16.4 months of patients with low combined score[39].

Inside MPM TME, Tregs play a significant part in immune modulation and tumor progression and are able to attenuate the activity of effector and helper T-cells[40].

Needham DJ et al. showed in murine MPM models that the depletion of intra-tumor Tregs with anti-CD25 monoclonal antibody injected directly into the tumors led to significantly reduced tumor growth, paving the way to new immunotherapeutic treatment strategies[41]. Chee SJ and colleagues observed that a higher number of $FOXP3^+$ T-cells was significantly

---

[37] A et al., "Phenotypic and Functional Analysis of Malignant Mesothelioma Tumor-Infiltrating Lymphocytes."
[38] Thapa et al., "OA08.05 Quantifying Tumour Infiltrating Lymphocytes (TILs) in Malignant Pleural Mesothelioma (MPM) -Defining the Hot, the Warm and the Cold Tumours."
[39] G et al., "Malignant Pleural Mesothelioma Immune Microenvironment and Checkpoint Expression: Correlation with Clinical-Pathological Features and Intratumor Heterogeneity over Time."
[40] S et al., "Regulatory T Cells and Immune Tolerance."
[41] DJ, JX, and MW, "Intra-Tumoural Regulatory T Cells: A Potential New Target in Cancer Immunotherapy."

associated with poorer survival in both epithelioid and non-epithelioid MPM patients[42].

Not only T cells but also B cells detain a role inside MPM TME.

Patil et al. performed both immunohistochemistry (IHC) and immune gene expression analysis and recognized three MPM subgroups: group 2 showed higher relative expression of B-cell and antigen presentation–related genes43. Interestingly, a preclinical work showed possible cytotoxic role activity of B cells against mesothelioma cells. In murine models of MPM authors demonstrated that, after intra tumor administration of agonist anti-CD40 antibody (Ab), the only tumor-infiltrating immune cell type that increased in number was the B cells. Their results suggest that the antitumor response induced by intra tumor anti-CD40 Ab involves mainly follicular (FO) B cells and not CD8+ T cells. CD40-activated splenic FO B cells mature into plasma cells that produce Abs directed at autoantigens overexpressed by mesothelioma cells and able to induce antibody-dependent cellular cytotoxicity (ADCC)[44].

An interest work analyzed the impact of immune cells phenotype inside TME on the outcome of patients affected by mesothelioma and they found that high $CD20^+$ counts, related to B cells infiltration, along with high $CD4^+$ cells and low $NP57^+$ counts (neutrophils), was associated with better prognosis in epithelioid MPM[45].

Taking into account immune check-points expression, it is well known that PD-L1 correlates with the sarcomatoid and biphasic histology[46]. Furthermore, Ghanim B et al. showed that patients with PD-L1 positive tumors (≥1%) had significantly shorter OS than patients with negative PD-

---

[42] SJ et al., "Evaluating the Effect of Immune Cells on the Outcome of Patients with Mesothelioma."
[43] NS et al., "Molecular and Histopathological Characterization of the Tumor Immune Microenvironment in Advanced Stage of Malignant Pleural Mesothelioma."
[44] C et al., "CD40-Activated B Cells Contribute to Mesothelioma Tumor Regression."
[45] SJ et al., "Evaluating the Effect of Immune Cells on the Outcome of Patients with Mesothelioma."
[46] S et al., "Shorter Survival in Malignant Pleural Mesothelioma Patients With High PD-L1 Expression Associated With Sarcomatoid or Biphasic Histology Subtype: A Series of 214 Cases From the Bio-MAPS Cohort."

L1 status and demonstrated a significant interaction of circulating C-reactive protein (CRP) with tumor PD-L1 expression, observing a very strong prognostic negative role of CPR in PD-L1 positive tumors but not in PD-L1 negative MPM[47].

Awad MM et al. correlated the lymphocyte subpopulations phenotype in tumor tissue of a cohort of MPM patients using both cyto-fluorimetry and IHC, with PD-L1 expression, suggesting that immunologic phenotypes in MPM might change based on PD-L1 status. PD-L1–positive tumors were characterized by a significantly higher proportion of proliferating $CD8^+$ T cells, a higher number of Tregs, and increased expression of PD-1 and TIM-3 on $CD4^+$ and $CD8^+$ T cells. Moreover, sarcomatoid and biphasic mesothelioma samples were significantly more likely to be PD-L1 positive and showed more infiltration with $CD3^+$ T cells[48].

Another immune check-point, CTLA4, has been investigated in MPM to restore anti-tumor immune cell activity, and combination of ipilimumab (an anti-CTLA 4 molecule) and nivolumab (anti PD1) has been approved by FDA as first line for MPM[49].

V-domain Ig-containing suppressor of T-cell activation (VISTA) is another immune checkpoint that inhibits anti-tumor immune responses and VISTA gene expression was reported to be higher in MPM than in all other cancer types mainly in epithelioid histotype, becoming a new potential target for mesothelioma immunotherapy. Muller S. and colleagues observed that IHC VISTA expression was related to better prognosis in MPM patients, independent of histotype[50].

---

[47] B et al., "Tumour Cell PD-L1 Expression Is Prognostic in Patients with Malignant Pleural Effusion: The Impact of C-Reactive Protein and Immune-Checkpoint Inhibition."
[48] MM et al., "Cytotoxic T Cells in PD-L1-Positive Malignant Pleural Mesotheliomas Are Counterbalanced by Distinct Immunosuppressive Factors."
[49] P et al., "First-Line Nivolumab plus Ipilimumab in Unresectable Malignant Pleural Mesothelioma (CheckMate 743): A Multicentre, Randomised, Open-Label, Phase 3 Trial."
[50] S et al., "V-Domain Ig-Containing Suppressor of T-Cell Activation (VISTA), a Potentially Targetable Immune Checkpoint Molecule, Is Highly Expressed in Epithelioid Malignant Pleural Mesothelioma."

Recently a new molecular classification based on a continuum score was proposed for MPM by Alcala N and colleagues[51]. They demonstrated that MPM prognosis is better explained by a continuous model, whose extremes show specific expression patterns of genes involved in angiogenesis and immune response.

The extremes of this continuum model detained specific molecular profiles: a "hot" subgroup, with high T-cells infiltration and high expression of immune checkpoints and pro-angiogenic genes, which showed a bad prognosis; a "cold" subgroup, with low T cells infiltration and high expression of pro-angiogenic genes, also related to bad prognosis; and another subgroup characterized by better prognosis, with high expression of VISTA and vascular endothelial growth factor receptor 2 (VEGFR2).

Since the immune system and angiogenic pathways interact with each other, they might better describe the heterogeneity of MPM when taken together into account. This might help researchers in the field to move beyond classic histological classification in the quest of new biomarkers in the era of immunotherapy and target therapy.

Tumor mutational burden (TMB), that quantifies the total number of somatic/acquired mutations per coding area of a tumor genome (Mut/Mb) harbored by tumor cells, has been deeply investigated as a biomarker of response to immunotherapy and FDA approved pembrolizumab for all solid tumors based on the KEYNOTE-158 study, which demonstrated durable responses in patients with a TMB ≥ 10 Mut/Mb[52]. A recent work showed that median TMB of 980 patients MPM was 1.74 Mut/Mb and that non-epithelioid and epithelioid MPM detained the same TMB (1.25 mut/mb vs 1.25 mut/mb, respectively)[53], confirming previous studies and

---

[51] N et al., "Redefining Malignant Pleural Mesothelioma Types as a Continuum Uncovers Immune-Vascular Interactions."
[52] A et al., "Association of Tumour Mutational Burden with Outcomes in Patients with Advanced Solid Tumours Treated with Pembrolizumab: Prospective Biomarker Analysis of the Multicohort, Open-Label, Phase 2 KEYNOTE-158 Study."
[53] Dagogo-Jack et al., "Comprehensive Molecular Profiling of Pleural Mesothelioma According to Histologic Subtype."

placing MPM within the group of low tumor mutational signature in human cancer. MPM is characterized by multiple structural chromosomal abnormalities that are not found with next generation sequencing (NGS) technique, partially explaining the unexpected low TMB detected in MPM, unusual for a cancer derived by exposure to environmental carcinogens and the subsequent inflammation. Mansfield and colleagues, using both a high-density array- comparative genomic hybridization and NGS, detected an higher number of genetic alterations, including copy number changes and all types of chromosomal rearrangements, than previously reported by only NGS. This study paves the way for a rethinking of the concept of MPM as a low TMB tumor, underlining the needed of further studies of the biology and pathogenesis of this rare and lethal cancer[54].

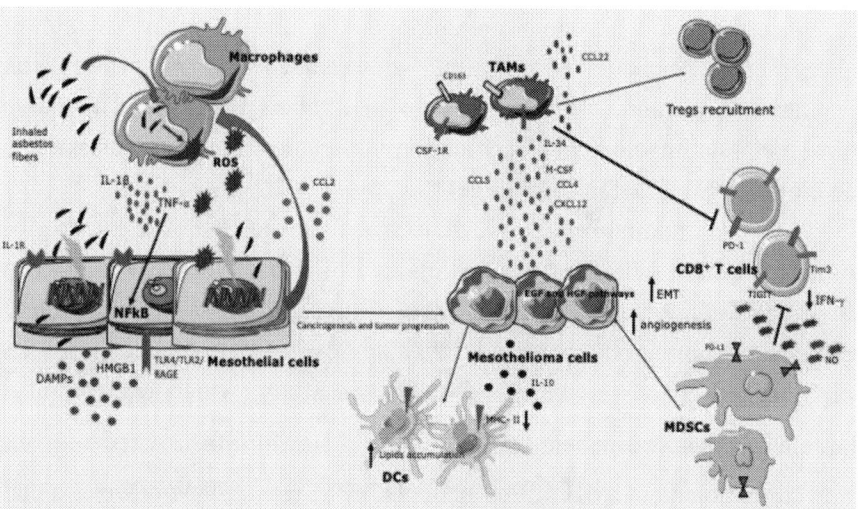

Figure 1. Asbestos fibers are inhaled deeply into the lung and penetrate the pleural space. Here, they interact with both mesothelial cells and inflammatory cells, mainly macrophages, leading to tissue damage, and local inflammation. Recruited macrophages phagocyte asbestos fibers but they are unable to digest them, therefore produce abundant reactive oxygen species (ROS).

---

[54] C and SM, "Molecular Characterization of Malignant Mesothelioma: Time for New Targets?"

Moreover, macrophages secrete proinflammatory mediators such as TNF-a and IL-1β, supporting carcinogenesis. IL-1β released by macrophages and its binding to IL-1R on mesothelial cells induce cell survival and proliferation, leading to malignant evolution. TNF-a released by macrophages promotes NF-kB pathway in mesothelial cells, supporting their survival to asbestos fibers. ROS lead to DNA damage in mesothelial cells, inducing necrotic cell death and the production and release of damage-associated molecular patterns (DAMPs) including High Mobility Group Box 1 protein (HMGB1), that, binding to TLR2, TLR4 and Advanced Glycation Endproducts (RAGE), promote mesothelial cells survival and malignant transformation.

Inside the tumor microenvironment (TME), tumor-associated macrophages (TAMs) play a key role. C–C chemokine ligand 4 (CCL4), C–C chemokine ligand 5 (CCL5) and C-X-C motif chemokine ligand 12 (CXCL12), secreted by MPM cells induce TAMs recruitment and activation, together with IL-34 and macrophage colony-stimulating factor (M-CSF), that binds its ligand colony stimulating factor-1 receptor (CSF-1R) on TAMs surface. TAMs are able to generate an immunosuppressive TME, recruiting and activating regulatory T cells (Tregs) and blocking $CD8^+T$ cells. TME of malignant pleural mesothelioma (MPM) also hosts myeloid-derived suppressor cells (MDSCs) that inhibit $CD8^+$ T cells activity also producing ROS and nitric oxide (NO) and reducing IFN-g synthesis. Mesothelioma Cells, by releasing immunosuppressive cytokines, such as IL-10, are able to suppress antigen-presentation activity of dendritic cells (DCs), reducing Major histocompatibility complex ii (MHC-II) expression, and inducing intracellular lipid accumulation that boost DCs dysfunction. Finally, T cells, MDSCs and TAMs express on their surfaces several immune checkpoint such as PD-1, PD-L1, TIM3, T-cell immunoreceptor with Ig and ITIM domains protein (TIGIT) that boost the immunosuppressive phenotype of MPM TME.

IMMUNE CHECK-POINT INHIBITORS

Brief History of Immunotherapy in Malignant Pleural Mesothelioma

Considering the numerous preclinical evidences that highlight the interaction between the immune system and MPM, immunotherapy has been trialed in this kind of patients over more than 25 years. The first evidence date back to 1990, when combinations of immunomodulators such as IFN-gamma and IL-2 began to be tested in patients with MPM with poor results[55]. In 1993, a study was published evaluating the association of IFN-alpha and doxorubicin in first-line setting[56]. This combination showed only modest activity in terms of objective response rate (ORR) and was associated with significant toxicity; therefore it was not recommended for the treatment of MPM. Later, in 1998, cytokine therapies emerged as treatments for solid tumors[57] and about MPM, a study investigated the effectiveness of intralesional GM-CSF infusion that produced a localized immune reaction. However, only a minority of patients had a response to the treatment[58]. Between 2006 and 2007, GM-CSF was tested in combination with autologous tumor cells as a vaccine for the treatment of several solid tumors, including MPM. In this context, vaccination with autologous MPM tumor cell lysate with GM-CSF induced tumor specific immunity in 32% of patients and was associated with stable disease but no major tumor regressions[59,60]. Other evidences supporting that MPM may be an immunogenic tumor is linked to occasional reports of

---

[55] Serke and Loddenkemper, "Therapeutische Optionen Beim Malignen Pleuramesotheliom."
[56] JW et al., "Interferon Alpha and Doxorubicin in Malignant Mesothelioma: A Phase II Study."
[57] BW et al., "Cytokine Gene Therapy or Infusion as Treatment for Solid Human Cancer."
[58] JA et al., "Intralesional Cytokine Therapy in Cancer: A Pilot Study of GM-CSF Infusion in Mesothelioma."
[59] S et al., "A Phase-I Trial Using a Universal GM-CSF-Producing and CD40L-Expressing Bystander Cell Line (GM.CD40L) in the Formulation of Autologous Tumor Cell-Based Vaccines for Cancer Patients with Stage IV Disease."
[60] A et al., "Recombinant GM-CSF plus Autologous Tumor Cells as a Vaccine for Patients with Mesothelioma."

spontaneous regression and serological evidence of immune responses, also reported in the early 2000s[61,62]. More recently, in 2010, an anti-TGFß monoclonal antibody was tested in patients with relapsed MPM and an antitumor humoral immunity was observed in almost half of the members, but it did not yield results in the outcome. Nevertheless, none of these treatments led to changes in clinical practice, mainly due to the logistical difficulties of local infusions and poor benefits.

Advent of Immune Checkpoint Inhibitors

The advent of PD-1/PD-L1 ICIs, both as single agents and in combination with chemotherapy and, more recently, ICIs combination, anti-PD-1 and anti-CTLA4, led to breakthrough therapeutic advances in many types of cancer, such as advanced non-small cell lung cancer (NSCLC), melanoma, renal cell carcinoma and others. About MPM, evidence from clinical trials of ICIs in this rare disease, suggests that such therapies may play a role as a treatment option for a proportion of patients with this cancer and in different settings.

Checkpoint Inhibitor within the Salvage Setting

Anti-CTLA4

The first clinical trials investigating ICIs in MPM were developed chronologically after the promising results of anti-CTLA4 in melanoma. Tremelimumab, an anti-CTLA4 antibody, was initially administered to patients with chemotherapy-resistant MPM in an open-label phase II trial. This study showed 7% partial responses (PR), 24% stable disease (SD),

---

[61] BW, C, and RA, "Localised Spontaneous Regression in Mesothelioma -- Possible Immunological Mechanism."

[62] C et al., "Serologic Responses in Patients with Malignant Mesothelioma: Evidence for Both Public and Private Specificities."

and 69% progressive disease (PD). The median PFS was 6.2 months and median OS 10.7 months[63]. Calabro et al. in another comparable study, substantially confirmed these results in the same patient setting. Similar PFS (6.2 months), OS (11.3 months) and ORR were observed[64].

The aforementioned PFS data and the proportion of patients with SD, led to the conduction of the DETERMINE trial. This was a double-blind, multicentric, placebo-controlled, phase 2b trial conducted in patients with unresectable pleural or peritoneal malignant mesothelioma who had progressed after one or two previous systemic treatments for advanced disease. Patients were randomized to receive tremelimumab or placebo every 4 weeks for 7 doses and every 12 weeks thereafter until a treatment protocol discontinuation criterion was met. The primary endpoint was OS in the intention-to-treat population, but unfortunately DETERMINE was a negative trial, with a hazard ratio of 0.92 for OS, and a median OS of 7.7 months (tremelimumab) vs. 7.3 months (placebo)[65]. Nevertheless, the rates of PR and SD were similar to the two previous studies, although more frequent imaging allowed investigators to determine progression at an earlier timepoint. It was concluded that there was no role for single-agent anti-CTLA4 antibody as a second-line or subsequent treatment in mesothelioma.

Anti-PD1

In 2017, the KEYNOTE-028 phase I trial was the first study testing a PD-1 inhibitor (pembrolizumab) in 25 MPM patients with a positive tumor PD-L1 IHC. The trial reported interesting results with a response rate of 20%, a disease control rate (DCR) of 72% with a median duration of

---

[63] L et al., "Tremelimumab for Patients with Chemotherapy-Resistant Advanced Malignant Mesothelioma: An Open-Label, Single-Arm, Phase 2 Trial."
[64] L et al., "Efficacy and Safety of an Intensified Schedule of Tremelimumab for Chemotherapy-Resistant Malignant Mesothelioma: An Open-Label, Single-Arm, Phase 2 Study."
[65] M et al., "Tremelimumab as Second-Line or Third-Line Treatment in Relapsed Malignant Mesothelioma (DETERMINE): A Multicentre, International, Randomised, Double-Blind, Placebo-Controlled Phase 2b Trial."

response of 12 months[66]. Another phase II study conducted at the University of Chicago suggested that single-agent pembrolizumab in the salvage setting had robust activity in PD-L1 unselected mesothelioma patients, with median OS of 11.5 months and increasing PD-L1 expression being associated with a trend towards a higher response rate and more durable PFS[67]. In light of these data, the first randomized study in patients with recurrent MPM was presented in 2019; ETOP PROMISE-meso, randomized patients to chemotherapy (gemcitabine or vinorelbine) versus pembrolizumab. The primary endpoint (PFS) was not met with a median PFS for pembrolizumab of 2.5 versus 3.4 months in the chemotherapy arm. Surprisingly, the response rate was significantly higher in the pembrolizumab arm (22%) compared to chemotherapy (6%) despite an equal PFS. The median OS was 10.7 months for patients in the pembrolizumab arm vs. 11.7 months for chemotherapy. To note, forty-five patients out of the chemotherapy arm crossed over to pembrolizumab after progression on chemotherapy[68]. Single agent nivolumab (another PD-1 inhibitor) was tested in several single arm phase II trials, in a randomized, non-comparative phase II study of nivolumab and nivolumab-ipilimumab and in placebo-controlled phase III trial. NivoMes was the first single-arm phase II study of nivolumab in 38 patients who had relapsed disease or progressed to chemotherapy regimen. Upon recruitment patients received nivolumab administered every 2 weeks for a maximum of 12 months or until disease progression or unacceptable toxicity. ORR of 24% was observed, but the median PFS was disappointing with only 2.6 months[69]. In 2018, the Japanese Ministry of Health, Labor and Welfare approved nivolumab as a salvage therapy in mesothelioma based on the results of the

---

[66] EW et al., "Clinical Safety and Activity of Pembrolizumab in Patients with Malignant Pleural Mesothelioma (KEYNOTE-028): Preliminary Results from a Non-Randomised, Open-Label, Phase 1b Trial."

[67] Desai et al., "OA08.03 Phase II Trial of Pembrolizumab (NCT02399371) In Previously-Treated Malignant Mesothelioma (MM): Final Analysis."

[68] S et al., "A Multicentre Randomised Phase III Trial Comparing Pembrolizumab versus Single-Agent Chemotherapy for Advanced Pre-Treated Malignant Pleural Mesothelioma: The European Thoracic Oncology Platform (ETOP 9-15) PROMISE-Meso Trial."

[69] J et al., "Programmed Death 1 Blockade With Nivolumab in Patients With Recurrent Malignant Pleural Mesothelioma."

MERIT trial[70]. This study showed an ORR of 26%, 67%, and 25% for epithelioid, sarcomatoid, and biphasic histologic subtypes, respectively. Median duration of response was 11.1 months with a 68% disease control rate. Median OS and PFS were 17.3 and 6.1 months, respectively. However, despite the promising results, the MERIT trial had some limitations. The small sample size of the trial and the early-phase design limits data robustness and reduces the potential for subgroup analyses. Moreover, the single-arm non-randomized design prevented any direct comparison with alternative treatment options in this disease setting. The third study evaluating nivolumab as a single agent was the MAPS-2. This prospective multi-center Phase II trial had randomized 125 MPM patients who had progressed upon receiving 1 or 2 prior treatment regimens. This non-comparative study contained two arms, and patients were randomly allocated to receive either nivolumab or nivolumab plus ipilimumab (anti CTLA-4). ORRs were 26–28% in the nivolumab plus ipilimumab arm and 19% in the nivolumab alone arm. Median OS data observed was 11.9 months for the single therapy and 15.9 months for the combination. The nivolumab monotherapy arm reported a median PFS of 4.0 months[71]. Most recently, the CONFIRM trial (phase III) randomized 332 patients with previously treated MPM to nivolumab or placebo. Nivolumab compared with placebo achieved the two co-primary endpoints with longer PFS (3.0 vs 1.8 months) and OS (9.2 vs. 6.6 months). Grade 3–4 treatment-related adverse events (TRAEs) were reported in 19% in the nivolumab arm and in 6.3% on the placebo arm[72]. Interestingly, PD-L1 expression had no bearing on OS, whereas epithelioid histology was found to have a significant survival advantage with a 12 month OS (40 vs. 26.7 months). Despite this, data from the Dutch expanded access program, suggest that in a real-world setting patients with recurrent MPM, nivolumab did not provide the same

---

[70] M et al., "Clinical Efficacy and Safety of Nivolumab: Results of a M Ulticenter, Op e n-Label, Single-a r m, Japanese Phase II Study in Mal i Gnant Pleural Meso t Helioma (MERIT)."
[71] A et al., "Nivolumab or Nivolumab plus Ipilimumab in Patients with Relapsed Malignant Pleural Mesothelioma (IFCT-1501 MAPS2): A Multicentre, Open-Label, Randomised, Non-Comparative, Phase 2 Trial."
[72] MJ et al., "Ipilimumab and Nivolumab in the Treatment of Recurrent Malignant Pleural Mesothelioma (INITIATE): Results of a Prospective, Single-Arm, Phase 2 Trial."

benefits as observed in clinical trials with worse ORR and a median OS of only 6.7 months[73].

Anti PD-L1

A Phase IB trial (JAVELIN) examined avelumab, a PD-L1 inhibitor, in 53 patients with unresectable mesothelioma that progressed after platinum and pemetrexed treatment. In the trial patients received avelumab, 10 mg/kg, every 2 weeks. This trial found that there was an acceptable safety profile, but the results in terms of OS, PFS and ORR were not robust: ORR was 9% (5 patients) with complete response in 1 patient and partial response in 4 patients. Median PFS was 4.1 months, and the 12-month PFS rate was 17.4%. Median OS was 10.7 months, and the median 12-month OS rate was 43.8%[74].

Combination of Checkpoint Inhibitors

Historically, the first study that evaluated the combination of ICIs was the MAPS-2. The results of this study were discussed in the previous section (non-comparative double arm, nivolumab and nivolumab + ipilimumab). The clinical activity of combination ipilimumab-nivolumab was also seen in the Dutch INITIATE trial with a response rate of 38% and a DCR of 68% at three months. However, the combination treatment was more toxic than using a single ICI with 94% of patients experienced an adverse event, but most side effects were easily managed and no grade 5 toxicity was observed. At the time of reporting, median OS had not yet been reached but was estimated, with 95% confidence, to exceed 12.7 months[75]. The NIBIT-Meso-1 study was an open-label, non-randomized study Phase II study to evaluate the safety and efficacy of another combination, durvalumab and tremelimumab. Forty patients were enrolled

---

[73] L et al., "Nivolumab in Pre-Treated Malignant Pleural Mesothelioma: Real-World Data from the Dutch Expanded Access Program."
[74] R et al., "Efficacy and Safety of Avelumab Treatment in Patients with Advanced Unresectable Mesothelioma: Phase 1b Results From the JAVELIN Solid Tumor Trial."
[75] L et al., "Tremelimumab Combined with Durvalumab in Patients with Mesothelioma (NIBIT-MESO-1): An Open-Label, Non-Randomised, Phase 2 Study."

after either refusing a first line platinum-based chemotherapy, or having disease progression following one line of platinum-based therapy for advanced MPM. Fair activity was observed with a median OS of 16.6 months (similar to the combination arm in the MAPS-2) and treatment-related toxicity was generally manageable and reversible[76].

Checkpoint Inhibitors within the First-Line Setting

The first human clinical trial of chemoimmunotherapy in MPM combined the CD40 activating antibody (CP- 870,893) with cisplatin and pemetrexed in a phase I clinical trial in patients who had not previously received any treatment for their disease. Chemotherapy was received in standard doses and CP-870,896 was received on day 8 of the cycle. Patients received up to six cycles of combined therapy and up to a further six cycles of CP-870,893 if the disease was responding or stable. In 15 treated patients, six reported a PR (40%) and nine patients reported a SD (53%), with a median OS of 16.5 months and three patients surviving beyond 30 months[77]. Subsequently, in 2018, the final results of a single-arm, phase 2 trial (DREAM) designed to determine the activity, safety and tolerability of durvalumab, cisplatin and pemetrexed as first line therapy in MPM were presented. This trial was a non-randomized trial, and 54 patients received durvalumab, cisplatin, and pemetrexed for a maximum of 6 cycles, followed by durvalumab every 3 weeks until progression, or a maximum total of 12 months. It has been reported that 1-year OS was 65% at a median follow-up of 14.4 months, an ORR of 48% by modified Response Evaluation Criteria in Solid Tumors (mRECIST), a median PFS of 6.9 months and finally a PFS at 6 months (PFS6) of 57%. This suggests that a triplet regimen of cisplatin-pemetrexed plus durvalumab might

---

[76] AK et al., "A Phase 1b Clinical Trial of the CD40-Activating Antibody CP-870,893 in Combination with Cisplatin and Pemetrexed in Malignant Pleural Mesothelioma."
[77] Zalcman et al., "Checkmate 743: A Phase 3, Randomized, Open-Label Trial of Nivolumab (Nivo) plus Ipilimumab (Ipi) vs Pemetrexed plus Cisplatin or Carboplatin as First-Line Therapy in Unresectable Pleural Mesothelioma."

induce promising tumor responses, and warrants extension into a Phase III clinical trial[78].

Combination of Checkpoint Inhibitors

Based on the encouraging activity of the ICI combination in the salvage setting, this strategy was tested in the first line setting. In fact, evidence derived from ongoing and recently published trials confirm that ICI combinations will be important new agents in the frontline setting for the management of MPM. In this context, a particularly relevant study was the CheckMate 743, on the basis of which the combination of nivolumab and ipilimumab was approved by the FDA in October 2020 and by European Medicines Agency (EMA) in April 2021 for previously untreated patients with unresectable or advanced MPM. The phase 3 CheckMate 743 trial, randomized 605 patients with unresectable MPM to receive either nivolumab and ipilimumab (303 patients) or platinum plus pemetrexed chemotherapy (302 patients). Notably, patients were not selected by histology or PD-L1 status. ICI significantly improved OS by 4 months compared to chemotherapy, with median OS of 18.1 versus 14.1 months, the 2-year OS was 41% and 27%, respectively, despite the fact that 20% of patients in the control arm received ICI at the time of progression. The difference in median OS was more pronounced in patients with non-epithelioid histology (18.1 *vs*. 8.8 months) and in PD-L1 positive (cut-off ≥1%) tumors (18.0 *vs*. 13.3). Of note, the proportion of grade 3–4 TRAEs were similar in both arms, in particular grade 3-4 TRAEs were reported in 91 (30%) of 300 patients treated with nivolumab plus ipilimumab and 91 (32%) of 284 treated with chemotherapy. Beyond the studies presented, it is important to underline that the topic of ICI and MPM is still open and numerous studies are currently underway summarized in Table 1.

---

[78] P et al., "First-Line Nivolumab plus Ipilimumab in Unresectable Malignant Pleural Mesothelioma (CheckMate 743): A Multicentre, Randomised, Open-Label, Phase 3 Trial."

Table 1. Ongoing clinical trials for immune check-point inhibitors in MPM patients

Status	Title	Trial Identifier	Treatment	Phase	Primary Objective	Patients enrolled	Type of solid tumor and setting
Recruiting	A Pilot Window-Of-Opportunity Study of the Anti-PD-1 Antibody Pembrolizumab in Patients With Resectable Malignant Pleural Mesothelioma	NCT02707666	Pembrolizumab + Cisplatin and Pemetrexed	1	Safety and gamma-Interferon Gene Expression profile (GEP) response	15	Advanced MPM, in first line
Recruiting	Pembrolizumab Plus Lenvatinib In Second Line and Third Line Malignant Pleural mesothelioma Patients	NCT04287829	Pembrolizumab + Lenvatinib	2	ORR	36	Advanced MPM, in Second Line and Third Line
Not yet recruiting	Pembrolizumab in Combination With Chemotherapy and Image-Guided Surgery for Malignant Pleural Mesothelioma (MPM)	NCT03760575	Pembrolizumab + Chemotherapy + image-Guided Surgery	1	Safety and tolerability	92	Perioperative setting
Recruiting	Nivolumab With Chemotherapy in Pleural Mesothelioma After Surgery	NCT04177953	Platinum based chemotherapy + Nivolumab	2	Time-to-next-treatment (TNT) and safety	92	MPM, adjuvant setting
Recruiting	Pembrolizumab With or Without Anetumab Ravtansine in Treating	NCT03126630	Pembrolizumab +/- Anetumab Ravtansine	1-2	Safety and tolerability	110	Advanced and pretreated MPM

Status	Title	Trial Identifier	Treatment	Phase	Primary Objective	Patients enrolled	Type of solid tumor and setting
Recruiting	MTG201 Plus Nivolumab in Patients With Relapsed Pleural Mesothelioma	NCT04013334	Nivolumab + MGT20	2	ORR	12	Advanced and pretreated MPM
Not yet recruiting	Neoadjuvant Toripalimab Combined With Chemotherapy in the Treatment of Malignant Pleural Mesothelioma	NCT04713761	Toripalimab + chemotherapy	2	Major pathologic response (MPR) and safety	15	MPM, neoadjuvant setting
Recruiting	A Study of Nivolumab and Chemotherapy Followed by Surgery for Mesothelioma	NCT04162015	Nivolumab + Chemotherapy	1	Number of patients going to operating room for surgical resection	35	MPM, neoadjuvant setting
Recruiting	Neoadjuvant Immune Checkpoint Blockade in Resectable Malignant Pleural Mesothelioma	NCT03918252	Nivolumab + Ipilimumab	1-2	Safety and Feasibility	30	MPM, neoadjuvant setting
Recruiting	Durvalumab With chemotherapy as First Line treAtment in Advanced Pleural Mesothelioma	NCT04334759	Chemotherapy +/- Durvalumab +	3	OS	480	Advanced MPM, in first line
	Patients With MPM						

Most of these have the objective of improving the survival of patients, focus on selecting the best ICI combination for each patient, as well incorporating ICI into the treatment strategy of resectable MPM.

OTHER IMMUNOTHERAPIES

Vaccines

In the last ten years, immunotherapy with vaccines has been identified as a therapeutic approach alternative to ICIs and potentially efficient against cancer cells. The mechanism being exploited is to address T-cell maturation against tumor-specific antigens (TSA) or tumor-associated antigens (TAA), that are processed by antigen-presenting cells (APCs). T-cells maturation occurs in the thymus and may be achieved indifferently against TSAs and TAAs, that represent two different groups of antigens. TSA are expressed only on cancer cells and are not present on normal tissues. In order to exploit TSAs as components of vaccine-based therapies, they need to derive from common and easily identifiable genetic alterations on cancer patients' tumor tissues. In addition to be addressed against TSAs, T lymphocytes may also react to common determinants that have been found both on cancer and normal cells, but are overexpressed on tumor tissue. Antigens whose epigenetic control or post-translational modifications may cause an overexpression on cancer cells surface membranes at an aberrant level are called tumor-associated antigens (TAA), such as p53. Thus, the mechanism to build anti-tumor vaccines is to identify potential TSA and TAA by tumor cells extracted from patient or cell cultures and deliver high concentrations of antigens in order to develop immune cells targeted against these antigens and enhance selectively specific immune response[79]. Vaccine-based immunotherapies have been investigated in different types of solid tumors: in a literature review, 8,1%

---

[79] MA, JA, and CW, "Antigens for Cancer Immunotherapy."

of cancer patients with a wide range of primitive tumor site treated with antigens derived from autologous or allogeneic tumor cells had an objective clinical response to immunotherapies, compared to 3,6% of those receiving molecularly defined (synthetic) antigens. No difference about response rate was seen between autologous and allogeneic tumor sources[80]. After exciting results of efficacy of ICIs against PD-1, PD-L1 and CTLA4 during the last years and their subsequent approvals in treatment of different solid tumors, it remains unanswered if tumor antigen-based therapy could in future play a role in this setting. In the last ten years, with technological advances in genomics and cancer immunotherapy, several preclinical and clinical trials have investigated different techniques to identify vaccine targets from autologous or allogeneic tumor cells and to produce a therapy personalized for the individual tumor mutation signatures. The first in-human studies have shown feasibility, safety and potential immunotherapeutic activity of vaccines on solid cancer patients[81]. About vaccine-based clinical trials in MPM patients, the SKOPOS trial is among the first ones[82]: it was a phase II, open-label and single arm study that investigated the immunological activity of the TroVax® vaccine in combination with first-line chemotherapy (pemetrexed-cisplatin) in patients with locally advanced or metastatic MPM. The TroVax® vaccine is a cancer vaccine composed of an attenuated vaccinia virus containing 5T4 glycoprotein gene that is widely expressed in all MPM subtypes. This vaccine demonstrated to induce 5T4-specific antibody and/or cellular immune responses in other types of solid tumors. By obtaining a humoral or cellular immune response on 95,6% of the 27 patients enrolled, the SKOPOS trial reached its primary endpoint.

The TroVax® vaccine showed acceptable safety and tolerability and a strong correlation between tumor-infiltrating CD8+ T cells and long

---

[80] MA, JA, and CW.
[81] U and Ö, "Personalized Vaccines for Cancer Immunotherapy."
[82] Lester et al., "A Single Centre Phase II Trial to Assess the Immunological Activity of TroVax® plus Pemetrexed/Cisplatin in Patients with Malignant Pleural Mesothelioma – the SKOPOS Trial."

survival was noted. Another clinical trial[83] investigated the immunogenicity of a vaccine composed by a synthetic peptide analog of the Wilms-tumor 1 (WT1) protein, that is overexpressed in MPM. The WT1-based vaccine was administered with adjuvants agents (Montanide and GM-CSF) in the treatment arm which comprised MPM patients after surgery and another treatment modality. The primary endpoint was 1-year PFS and the control arm received Montanide and GM-CSF alone, not being this phase II study designed or powered for comparison between the arms. In addition to confirmation of well-tolerability and safety, the use of analog WT1 peptide vaccine was associated with a not-statistically significant increase in PFS and OS. Powell et al.[84] conducted a phase II study whose primary endpoint was to increase tumor specific immunity in MPM patients by administering a vaccine manufactured from autologous tumor cell lysate (obtained from surgically resected tumor) plus recombinant GM-CSF. Twenty-two patients with stage III or IV MPM were enrolled and none of them received prior cytotoxic therapy or immunotherapy. Of these seven (32%) developed at least one type of anti-MPM immune response, revealed by positivity of delayed type hypersensitivity skin testing or altered pattern of antibody reactivity by western blotting. The vaccine was safe and associated with SD in 46% of cases but not with tumor objective responses. This study showed a 1-year and 2-year survival rates of 50% and 27% respectively, comparable to chemotherapy results, despite that a direct comparison is not feasible.

---

[83] MG et al., "A Randomized Phase II Trial of Adjuvant Galinpepimut-S, WT-1 Analogue Peptide Vaccine, After Multimodality Therapy for Patients with Malignant Pleural Mesothelioma."

[84] Powell et al., "Recombinant GM-CSF plus Autologous Tumor Cells as a Vaccine for Patients with Mesothelioma."

Table 2. Ongoing clinical trials for vaccine-based immunotherapy in MPM patients

Status	Title	Trial Identifier	Treatment	Phase	Primary Objective(s)	Patients enrolled	Type of solid tumor and setting
Active, not recruiting	A Randomised Phase II Open-label Study With a Phase Ib Safety lead-in Cohort of ONCOS-102, an Immune-priming GM-CSF Coding Oncolytic Adenovirus, and Pemetrexed/Cisplatin in Patients With Unresectable Malignant Pleural Mesothelioma	NCT02879669	pemetrexed/cisplatin +/- ONCOS-102 and cyclophosphamide	1; 2	Safety and tolerability	31	Advanced MPM, in first or subsequent line
Recruiting	Nivolumab and Ipilimumab +/- UV1 Vaccination as Second Line Treatment in Patients With Malignant Mesothelioma (NIPU)	NCT04300244	Nivolumab + ipilimumab +/-UV1 vaccine + leukine	2	PFS	118	Advanced MPM, after first line chemotherapy
Recruiting	Using a Targeted Cancer Vaccine (Galinpepimut-S) With Immunotherapy (Nivolumab) in Mesothelioma	NCT04040231	Galinpepimut-S +Nivolumab + Sargramostim	1	Maximum tolerated dose	10	Advanced and pretreated MPM and Wilms Tumor
Recruiting	Poly-ICLC (Hiltonol®) Vaccine In Malignant Pleural Mesothelioma	NCT04525859	Poly-ICLC	1; 1b	Safety and tolerability	19	MPM, neoadjuvant setting
Recruiting	First-in-human Study of S-588210 (S-488210+S-488211)	NCT04316689	S-488210 + S-488211	1	Safety and tolerability	10	Advanced and pretreated MPM and other solid tumors

More recently, Kennedy et al.[85] developed a murine model of MPM through transduction of a mesothelioma cell line with the mesothelin gene, that encodes for a surface antigen overexpressed in MPM and represents a potential immunothera-peutic target. Then, it was created a recombinant Listeria monocytogenes-based vaccine for mesothelin, able to induce an immune antitumor response and to induce epitope spreading in several malignant neoplasms. It was demonstrated that tumor growth was significantly inhibited in mice inoculated with this vaccine prior to or concurrently with cancer cell inoculation; differently mesothelin-expressing Listeria vaccine was not efficient against established primary tumors.

Furthermore, it was noted that cytoreductive surgery plays a role in reducing systemic tumor-related immunosuppression and may be costimulatory to Listeria-based vaccine. A subsequent phase Ib clinical trial[86] involved unresectable MPM patients receiving a live-attenuated Listeria monocytogenes engineered to express mesothelin in combination with pemetrexed/cisplatin chemotherapy. The treatment resulted safe and induced a significant objective tumor response (89%), with a tumor size reduction in 31% of cases occurring prior to chemotherapy infusion. This combination was able to induce changes of immune cells infiltrating the local tumor microenvironment. A potential obstacle to efficacy of monotherapy with antitumor vaccines may be the loss of a single antigen target or the intratumoral heterogeneity, or other mechanisms of the immune escape[87]. From these results, it can be argued that vaccine-based immunotherapy integrated with other types of treatment should be considered part of a "multidisciplinary" therapy protocol. Table 2 summarizes the ongoing clinical trials involving MPM patients receiving vaccine-based immunotherapy.

---

[85] GT et al., "Surgical Cytoreduction Restores the Antitumor Efficacy of a Listeria Monocytogenes Vaccine in Malignant Pleural Mesothelioma."
[86] Hassan et al., "Clinical Response of Live-Attenuated, Listeria Monocytogenes Expressing Mesothelin (CRS-207) with Chemotherapy in Patients with Malignant Pleural Mesothelioma."
[87] Cebon, "Perspective: Cancer Vaccines in the Era of Immune Checkpoint Blockade."

Cellular Immunotherapy

A new therapeutic opportunity for MPM patients derived from studies regarding stimulation of immune response against tumor cells by cellular therapy[88,89]. From the basis of preclinical studies, there have been identified chimeric antigen receptor T (CAR-T) cells, that are genetically engineered T-cells extracted from the patient and triggered to produce tumor-specific CAR. After reintroducing altered T cells into cancer patients, CAR-T are able to specifically recognize and bind a target on tumor cell surface and to deliver a T-cell activating signal[90]. They have been largely studied and approved for hematological malignancies and recently preclinical and clinical trials focused on their use on solid tumors, such as melanoma, glioblastoma and ovarian cancer. Looking at MPM, Adusumilli et al.[91] conducted a phase I trial using the intrapleural administration of a CD28-costimulated mesothelin CAR with the Icaspase-9 safety gene (IcasM28z). No related toxicity emerged and CAR T-cell therapy combined with anti-PD1 agents showed encouraging clinical outcomes in 19 MPM patients, especially 2 complete responses (CR) and 5 PR. Another clinical trial employed FAP-specific CD8+ re-directed T cells in MPM patients with pleural effusion[92], administered intrapleurally. Fibroblast activation protein (FAP) is overexpressed in all three major MPM subtypes. Results showed a good tolerance of treatment and a persistence of CAR-T cells in the peripheral blood. From results showed in mouse models, it seems that CAR-T cells and anti-PD1/PD-L1 inhibition therapy may mutually strengthen their potency, leading to a potential

---

[88] Gray and Mutti, "Immunotherapy for Mesothelioma: A Critical Review of Current Clinical Trials and Future Perspectives."
[89] SG, "Emerging Avenues in Immunotherapy for the Management of Malignant Pleural Mesothelioma."
[90] Srivastava and Riddell, "CAR T Cell Therapy: Challenges to Bench-to-Bedside Efficacy."
[91] Adusumilli et al., "Abstract CT036: A Phase I Clinical Trial of Malignant Pleural Disease Treated with Regionally Delivered Autologous Mesothelin-Targeted CAR T Cells: Safety and Efficacy."
[92] U et al., "Re-Directed T Cells for the Treatment of Fibroblast Activation Protein (FAP)-Positive Malignant Pleural Mesothelioma (FAPME-1)."

combination able to overcome resistance to immune monotherapy[93]. Moreover, several trials investigated the administration of DCs in advanced MPM patients. DCs as an immunotherapeutic approach derived from autologous CD14+ monocytes or CD34+ hematopoietic progenitors and are isolated from patients. They are exposed to autologous or allogenic tumor lysate and then can be loaded and activated with different types of tumor antigens. By administration in MPM patients, DCs showed to stimulate an anti-tumor immune response, involving both cytotoxic T lymphocytes and CD4+ T cells[94]. In the 2010s, first studies used autologous tumor lysate, demonstrating that DCs loaded with these antigens are well-tolerated in humans and may induce a specific and immune-mediated cytotoxic activity against autologous tumor cells[95]. Aerts et al.[96] showed that DC therapy with allogeneic tumor cell lysate is effective in a murine model and then they reproduce a similar treatment on MPM patients enrolled in a phase I study, leading to conclusion that DCs therapy is safe and feasibile also on humans. Beyond the small number of patients enrolled, the median PFS resulted 8.8 months and median OS was not reached at a median follow-up of 22.8 months. Promising results emerged also from an analysis on long-term follow-up of MPM patients enrolled in 3 phase I/II trials and treated with DCs therapy: an OS at 2 years of 55.2% e at 5 years of 20.7% was observed[97]. From these evidences, MPM patients are[98] currently recruited in a phase II/III trial with the aim to assess the potential advantage on OS of DCs (MesoPher) as maintenance therapy after chemotherapy. To extend clinical efficacy of

---

[93] L et al., "Human CAR T Cells with Cell-Intrinsic PD-1 Checkpoint Blockade Resist Tumor-Mediated Inhibition."
[94] A et al., "Antitumour Dendritic Cell Vaccination in a Priming and Boosting Approach."
[95] JP et al., "Consolidative Dendritic Cell-Based Immunotherapy Elicits Cytotoxicity against Malignant Mesothelioma."
[96] JGJV et al., "Autologous Dendritic Cells Pulsed with Allogeneic Tumor Cell Lysate in Mesothelioma: From Mouse to Human."
[97] DW et al., "Long-Term Follow-Up of Mesothelioma Patients Treated with Dendritic Cell Therapy in Three Phase I/II Trials."
[98] RA et al., "A Multicenter, Randomized, Phase II/III Study of Dendritic Cells Loaded with Allogeneic Tumor Cell Lysate (MesoPher) in Subjects with Mesothelioma as Maintenance Therapy after Chemotherapy: DENdritic Cell Immunotherapy for Mesothelioma (DENIM) Trial."

DCs on long-term, some combination strategies with chemotherapy, radiotherapy and immune checkpoint inhibitors have been studied[99]. Through induction of epitope spreading and stimulation of specific T cells against tumor antigens, the efficacy of DCs may be potentiated by activation of different molecular pathways of immune response. For example, cyclophosphamide in addition to autologous tumor lysate-pulsed DCs demonstrated to reduce circulating levels of regulatory T cells and to achieve a radiographic disease control in MPM patients, resulting in a potentially safe and efficient combination therapy[100]. Among ongoing studies, a phase 1/2 trial is investigating the combination of platinum/pemetrexed-based chemotherapy and DCs loaded with mesothelioma-associated tumor antigen WT1 in advanced MPM patients. The primary objective is feasibility and safety of the chemoimmunotherapy and the induction of systemic and local immunogenicity will be analyzed (ClinicalTrials.gov Identifier: NCT02649829). Also the approach of combination of two kinds of immunotherapy may provide interesting results: in a phase 1b trial (ClinicalTrials.gov Identifier: NCT03546426), patients with diagnosis of PD-L1 advanced MPM who have failed to standard therapies will be candidates to receive pembrolizumab in association with DCs loaded with autologous tumor homogenate and Interleukin-2. In addition to safety as primary objective, it will also explore the ability to induce PD-L1 expression on tumor tissues and to enhance the efficacy of ICIs. From these evidences, it appears clear that other kinds of immunotherapeutic approaches are feasible besides the blockade of PD-1/PD-L1 and CTLA4 axis. Immunotherapies based on vaccines or cellular therapy have demonstrated their safety and good tolerance in humans, also in MPM patients, whose treatment options in advanced settings still remain severely limited. Current studies are focusing on combination systemic treatments, in order to enhance the immunologic activity and to overcome

---

[99] van Gulijk et al., "Combination Strategies to Optimize Efficacy of Dendritic Cell-Based Immunotherapy."
[100] R et al., "Extended Tumor Control after Dendritic Cell Vaccination with Low-Dose Cyclophosphamide as Adjuvant Treatment in Patients with Malignant Pleural Mesothelioma."

the innate and acquired resistance, and should in future significantly improve MPM patient prognosis.

CONCLUSION

First positive results from trials investigating ICIs in MPM patients have led to a paradigm shift and sharply revamped the enthusiasm around immunotherapy options for this orphan disease. The potential to combine ICIs with other immunotherapies, as well as targeted agents and old-school chemotherapy is currently explored and expectations are now high that this will lead to a plethora of new treatment options and eventually to cure some mesothelioma patients. A new era is hopefully coming in which clinical scientists will be finally able to talk about treatment sequences with their MPM patients. In order to achieve that, clinical research should be strongly coupled with translational investigations, in the conduction of well-designed, biomarker-driven clinical trials, which should always take into account the rare incidence of this cancer entity. In fact, only acknowledging intra and inter-patient heterogeneity, by the integration of multiple tumor and patient parameters, will enable identification of MPM patients who are more likely to derive clinical benefit and ensure further development of immunotherapy drugs in this setting.

REFERENCES

Adusumilli, Prasad S, Marjorie G Zauderer, Valerie W Rusch, Roisin E O'Cearbhaill, Amy Zhu, Daniel A Ngai, Erin McGee, et al. "Abstract CT036: A Phase I Clinical Trial of Malignant Pleural Disease Treated with Regionally Delivered Autologous Mesothelin-Targeted CAR T Cells: Safety and Efficacy." *Cancer Research* 79, no. 13 Supplement (July 1, 2019): CT036–CT036. https://doi.org/10.1158/1538-7445.AM2019-CT036.

Aerts, JGJV, de Goeje PL, Cornelissen R, Kaijen-Lambers MEH, Bezemer K, van der Leest CH, Mahaweni NM, et al. "Autologous Dendritic Cells Pulsed with Allogeneic Tumor Cell Lysate in Mesothelioma: From Mouse to Human." *Clinical Cancer Research: An Official Journal of the American Association for Cancer Research* 24, no. 4 (December 12, 2017): 766–76. https://doi.org/10.1158/1078-0432.CCR-17-2522.

Aggarwal, C, and Albelda SM. "Molecular Characterization of Malignant Mesothelioma: Time for New Targets?" *Cancer Discovery* 8, no. 12 (December 1, 2018): 1507–10. https://doi.org/10.1158/2159-8290.CD-18-1181.

Alcala, N, Mangiante L, Le-Stang N, Gustafson CE, Boyault S, Damiola F, Alcala K, et al. "Redefining Malignant Pleural Mesothelioma Types as a Continuum Uncovers Immune-Vascular Interactions." *EBioMedicine* 48 (October 1, 2019): 191–202. https://doi.org/10.1016/J.EBIOM.2019.09.003.

Alley, EW, Lopez J, Santoro A, Morosky A, Saraf S, Piperdi B, and van Brummelen E. "Clinical Safety and Activity of Pembrolizumab in Patients with Malignant Pleural Mesothelioma (KEYNOTE-028): Preliminary Results from a Non-Randomised, Open-Label, Phase 1b Trial." *The Lancet. Oncology* 18, no. 5 (May 1, 2017): 623–30. https://doi.org/10.1016/S1470-2045(17) 30169-9.

Awad, MM, Jones RE, Liu H, Lizotte PH, Ivanova EV, Kulkarni M, Herter-Sprie GS, et al. "Cytotoxic T Cells in PD-L1-Positive Malignant Pleural Mesotheliomas Are Counterbalanced by Distinct Immunosuppressive Factors." *Cancer Immunology Research* 4, no. 12 (December 1, 2016): 1038–48. https://doi.org/10.1158/2326-6066.CIR-16-0171.

Baas, P, Scherpereel A, Nowak AK, Fujimoto N, Peters S, Tsao AS, Mansfield AS, et al. "First-Line Nivolumab plus Ipilimumab in Unresectable Malignant Pleural Mesothelioma (CheckMate 743): A Multicentre, Randomised, Open-Label, Phase 3 Trial." *Lancet (London, England)* 397, no. 10272 (January 30, 2021): 375–86. https://doi.org/10.1016/S0140-6736(20)32714-8.

Belderbos, RA, Baas P, Berardi R, Cornelissen R, Fennell DA, van Meerbeeck JP, Scherpereel A, Vroman H, and Aerts JGJV. "A Multicenter, Randomized, Phase II/III Study of Dendritic Cells Loaded with Allogeneic Tumor Cell Lysate (MesoPher) in Subjects with Mesothelioma as Maintenance Therapy after Chemotherapy: DENdritic Cell Immunotherapy for Mesothelioma (DENIM) Trial." *Translational Lung Cancer Research* 8, no. 3 (June 1, 2019): 280–85. https://doi.org/10.21037/TLCR.2019.05.05.

Blondy, T, d'Almeida SM, Briolay T, Tabiasco J, Meiller C, Chéné AL, Cellerin L, et al. "Involvement of the M-CSF/IL-34/CSF-1R Pathway in Malignant Pleural Mesothelioma." *Journal for Immunotherapy of Cancer* 8, no. 1 (June 1, 2020). https://doi.org/10.1136/JITC-2019-000182.

Brosseau, S, Danel C, Scherpereel A, Mazières J, Lantuejoul S, Margery J, Greillier L, et al. "Shorter Survival in Malignant Pleural Mesothelioma Patients With High PD-L1 Expression Associated With Sarcomatoid or Biphasic Histology Subtype: A Series of 214 Cases From the Bio-MAPS Cohort." *Clinical Lung Cancer* 20, no. 5 (September 1, 2019): e564–75. https://doi.org/10.1016/J.CLLC.2019.04.010.

Bruno, A, Mortara L, Baci D, Noonan DM, and Albini A. "Myeloid Derived Suppressor Cells Interactions With Natural Killer Cells and Pro-Angiogenic Activities: Roles in Tumor Progression." *Frontiers in Immunology* 10 (2019): 771. https://doi.org/10.3389/FIMMU.2019.00771.

Calabrò, L, Morra A, Fonsatti E, Cutaia O, Amato G, Giannarelli D, Di Giacomo AM, et al. "Tremelimumab for Patients with Chemotherapy-Resistant Advanced Malignant Mesothelioma: An Open-Label, Single-Arm, Phase 2 Trial." *The Lancet. Oncology* 14, no. 11 (October 2013): 1104–11. https://doi.org/10.1016/S1470-2045(13)70381-4.

Calabrò, L, Morra A, Fonsatti E, Cutaia O, Fazio C, Annesi D, Lenoci M, et al. "Efficacy and Safety of an Intensified Schedule of Tremelimumab for Chemotherapy-Resistant Malignant Mesothelioma: An Open-Label, Single-Arm, Phase 2 Study." *The Lancet. Respiratory*

Medicine 3, no. 4 (April 1, 2015): 301–9. https://doi.org/10.1016/S2213-2600(15)00092-2.

Calabrò, L, Morra A, Giannarelli D, Amato G, D'Incecco A, Covre A, Lewis A, et al. "Tremelimumab Combined with Durvalumab in Patients with Mesothelioma (NIBIT-MESO-1): An Open-Label, Non-Randomised, Phase 2 Study." *The Lancet. Respiratory Medicine* 6, no. 6 (June 1, 2018): 451–60. https://doi.org/10.1016/S2213-2600(18)30151-6.

Cantini, L, Belderbos RA, Gooijer CJ, Dumoulin DW, Cornelissen R, Baart S, Burgers JA, Baas P, and Aerts JGJV. "Nivolumab in Pre-Treated Malignant Pleural Mesothelioma: Real-World Data from the Dutch Expanded Access Program." *Translational Lung Cancer Research* 9, no. 4 (August 1, 2020): 1169–79. https://doi.org/10.21037/TLCR-19-686.

Cantini, L, Pecci F, Hurkmans DP, Belderbos RA, Lanese A, Copparoni C, Aerts S, et al. "High-Intensity Statins Are Associated with Improved Clinical Activity of PD-1 Inhibitors in Malignant Pleural Mesothelioma and Advanced Non-Small Cell Lung Cancer Patients." *European Journal of Cancer (Oxford, England : 1990)* 144 (February 1, 2021): 41–48. https://doi.org/10.1016/J.EJCA.2020.10.031.

Carbone, M, and Yang H. "Molecular Pathways: Targeting Mechanisms of Asbestos and Erionite Carcinogenesis in Mesothelioma." *Clinical Cancer Research : An Official Journal of the American Association for Cancer Research* 18, no. 3 (February 1, 2012): 598–604. https://doi.org/10.1158/1078-0432.CCR-11-2259.

Cebon, Jonathan. "Perspective: Cancer Vaccines in the Era of Immune Checkpoint Blockade." *Mammalian Genome* 29, no. 11–12 (December 1, 2018): 703–13. https://doi.org/10.1007/S00335-018-9786-Z.

Chee, SJ, Lopez M, Mellows T, Gankande S, Moutasim KA, Harris S, Clarke J, Vijayanand P, Thomas GJ, and Ottensmeier CH. "Evaluating the Effect of Immune Cells on the Outcome of Patients with Mesothelioma." *British Journal of Cancer* 117, no. 9 (2017): 1341–48. https://doi.org/10.1038/BJC.2017.269.

Chéné, AL, d'Almeida S, Blondy T, Tabiasco J, Deshayes S, Fonteneau JF, Cellerin L, Delneste Y, Grégoire M, and Blanquart C. "Pleural Effusions from Patients with Mesothelioma Induce Recruitment of Monocytes and Their Differentiation into M2 Macrophages." *Journal of Thoracic Oncology: Official Publication of the International Association for the Study of Lung Cancer* 11, no. 10 (2016): 1765–73. https://doi.org/10.1016/J.JTHO.2016.06.022.

Cherkassky, L, Morello A, Villena-Vargas J, Feng Y, Dimitrov DS, Jones DR, Sadelain M, and Adusumilli PS. "Human CAR T Cells with Cell-Intrinsic PD-1 Checkpoint Blockade Resist Tumor-Mediated Inhibition." *The Journal of Clinical Investigation* 126, no. 8 (August 1, 2016): 3130–44. https://doi.org/10.1172/JCI83092.

Chu, GJ, van Zandwijk N, and Rasko JEJ. "The Immune Microenvironment in Mesothelioma: Mechanisms of Resistance to Immunotherapy." *Frontiers in Oncology* 9 (December 6, 2019). https://doi.org/10.3389/FONC.2019.01366.

Cornelissen, R, Hegmans JP, Maat AP, Kaijen-Lambers ME, Bezemer K, Hendriks RW, Hoogsteden HC, and Aerts JG. "Extended Tumor Control after Dendritic Cell Vaccination with Low-Dose Cyclophosphamide as Adjuvant Treatment in Patients with Malignant Pleural Mesothelioma." *American Journal of Respiratory and Critical Care Medicine* 193, no. 9 (May 1, 2016): 1023–31. https://doi.org/10.1164/RCCM.201508-1573OC.

Cornelissen, R, Lievense LA, Maat AP, Hendriks RW, Hoogsteden HC, Bogers AJ, Hegmans JP, and Aerts JG. "Ratio of Intratumoral Macrophage Phenotypes Is a Prognostic Factor in Epithelioid Malignant Pleural Mesothelioma." *PloS One* 9, no. 9 (September 5, 2014). https://doi.org/10.1371/JOURNAL.PONE.0106742.

Curiel, TJ, Coukos G, Zou L, Alvarez X, Cheng P, Mottram P, Evdemon-Hogan M, et al. "Specific Recruitment of Regulatory T Cells in Ovarian Carcinoma Fosters Immune Privilege and Predicts Reduced Survival." *Nature Medicine* 10, no. 9 (September 2004): 942–49. https://doi.org/10.1038/NM1093.

Dagogo-Jack, Ibiayi, Russell Madison, Douglas A Mata, Alexa Betzig Schrock, Tyler Janovitz, Brennan Decker, Richard SP Huang, et al. *Comprehensive Molecular Profiling of Pleural Mesothelioma According to Histologic Subtype.* Https://Doi.Org/10.1200/JCO. 2021.39.15_suppl.8555 39, no. 15_suppl (May 28, 2021): 8555–8555. https://doi.org/10.1200/JCO.2021.39.15_SUPPL.8555.

Davidson, JA, Musk AW, Wood BR, Morey S, Ilton M, Yu LL, Drury P, Shilkin K, and Robinson BW. "Intralesional Cytokine Therapy in Cancer: A Pilot Study of GM-CSF Infusion in Mesothelioma." *Journal of Immunotherapy* (Hagerstown, Md.: 1997) 21, no. 5 (1998): 389. https://doi.org/10.1097/00002371-199809000-00007.

Davies, S, Beckenkamp A, and Buffon A. "CD26 a Cancer Stem Cell Marker and Therapeutic Target." *Biomedicine & Pharmacotherapy = Biomedecine & Pharmacotherapie* 71 (April 1, 2015): 135–38. https://doi.org/10.1016/J.BIOPHA.2015.02.031.

Desai, A, T Karrison, B Rose, Y Tan, B Hill, E Pemberton, C Straus, T Seiwert, and HL Kindler. "OA08.03 Phase II Trial of Pembrolizumab (NCT02399371) In Previously-Treated Malignant Mesothelioma (MM): Final Analysis." *Journal of Thoracic Oncology* 13, no. 10 (October 1, 2018): S339. https://doi.org/10.1016/J.JTHO.2018.08.277.

Dessureault, S, Noyes D, Lee D, Dunn M, Janssen W, Cantor A, Sotomayor E, Messina J, and Antonia SJ. "A Phase-I Trial Using a Universal GM-CSF-Producing and CD40L-Expressing Bystander Cell Line (GM.CD40L) in the Formulation of Autologous Tumor Cell-Based Vaccines for Cancer Patients with Stage IV Disease." *Annals of Surgical Oncology* 14, no. 2 (February 2007): 869–84. https://doi.org/10.1245/S10434-006-9196-4.

Disselhorst, MJ, Quispel-Janssen J, Lalezari F, Monkhorst K, de Vries JF, van der Noort V, Harms E, Burgers S, and Baas P. "Ipilimumab and Nivolumab in the Treatment of Recurrent Malignant Pleural Mesothelioma (INITIATE): Results of a Prospective, Single-Arm, Phase 2 Trial." *The Lancet. Respiratory Medicine* 7, no. 3 (March 1, 2019): 260–70. https://doi.org/10.1016/S2213-2600(18)30420-X.

Dumoulin, DW, Cornelissen R, Bezemer K, Baart SJ, and Aerts JGJV. "Long-Term Follow-Up of Mesothelioma Patients Treated with Dendritic Cell Therapy in Three Phase I/II Trials." *Vaccines* 9, no. 5 (May 1, 2021). https://doi.org/10.3390/VACCINES9050525.

Fennell, D, C Ottensmeier, R Califano, G Hanna, S Ewings, K Hill, S Wilding, et al. "PS01.11 Nivolumab Versus Placebo in Relapsed Malignant Mesothelioma: The CONFIRM Phase 3 Trial." *Journal of Thoracic Oncology* 16, no. 3 (March 1, 2021): S62. https://doi.org/10.1016/J.JTHO.2021.01.323.

Gardner, JK, Mamotte CD, Patel P, Yeoh TL, Jackaman C, and Nelson DJ. "Mesothelioma Tumor Cells Modulate Dendritic Cell Lipid Content, Phenotype and Function." *PloS One* 10, no. 4 (April 17, 2015). https://doi.org/10.1371/JOURNAL.PONE.0123563.

Ghanim, B, Rosenmayr A, Stockhammer P, Vogl M, Celik A, Bas A, Kurul IC, et al. "Tumour Cell PD-L1 Expression Is Prognostic in Patients with Malignant Pleural Effusion: The Impact of C-Reactive Protein and Immune-Checkpoint Inhibition." *Scientific Reports* 10, no. 1 (December 1, 2020). https://doi.org/10.1038/S41598-020-62813-2.

Gray, Steven G, and Luciano Mutti. "Immunotherapy for Mesothelioma: A Critical Review of Current Clinical Trials and Future Perspectives." *Translational Lung Cancer Research* 9, no. Suppl 1 (February 1, 2020): S100. https://doi.org/10.21037/TLCR.2019.11.23.

Gray. SG, "Emerging Avenues in Immunotherapy for the Management of Malignant Pleural Mesothelioma." *BMC Pulmonary Medicine* 21, no. 1 (December 1, 2021). https://doi.org/10.1186/S12890-021-01513-7.

Gulijk, Mandy van, Floris Dammeijer, Joachim GJV Aerts, and Heleen Vroman. "Combination Strategies to Optimize Efficacy of Dendritic Cell-Based Immunotherapy." *Frontiers in Immunology* 9 (December 5, 2018): 2759. https://doi.org/10.3389/FIMMU.2018.02759.

H, Yang, Testa JR, and Carbone M. "Mesothelioma Epidemiology, Carcinogenesis, and Pathogenesis." *Current Treatment Options in Oncology* 9, no. 2–3 (2008): 147–57. https://doi.org/10.1007/S11864-008-0067-Z.

Harari, A, Graciotti M, Bassani-Sternberg M, and Kandalaft LE. "Antitumour Dendritic Cell Vaccination in a Priming and Boosting Approach." *Nature Reviews. Drug Discovery* 19, no. 9 (September 1, 2020): 635–52. https://doi.org/10.1038/S41573-020-0074-8.

Hassan, R, Thomas A, Nemunaitis JJ, Patel MR, Bennouna J, Chen FL, Delord JP, et al. "Efficacy and Safety of Avelumab Treatment in Patients With Advanced Unresectable Mesothelioma: Phase 1b Results From the JAVELIN Solid Tumor Trial." *JAMA Oncology* 5, no. 3 (March 1, 2019): 351–57. https://doi.org/10.1001/JAMAONCOL.2018.5428.

Hassan, Raffit, Evan Alley, Hedy Kindler, Scott Antonia, Thierry Jahan, Somayeh Honarmand, Nitya Nair, et al. "Clinical Response of Live-Attenuated, Listeria Monocytogenes Expressing Mesothelin (CRS-207) with Chemotherapy in Patients with Malignant Pleural Mesothelioma." *Clinical Cancer Research* 25, no. 19 (October 1, 2019): 5787–98. https://doi.org/10.1158/1078-0432.CCR-19-0070.

Hegmans, JP, Veltman JD, Lambers ME, de Vries IJ, Figdor CG, Hendriks RW, Hoogsteden HC, Lambrecht BN, and Aerts JG. "Consolidative Dendritic Cell-Based Immunotherapy Elicits Cytotoxicity against Malignant Mesothelioma." *American Journal of Respiratory and Critical Care Medicine* 181, no. 12 (June 15, 2010): 1383–90. https://doi.org/10.1164/RCCM.200909-1465OC.

Horio, D, Minami T, Kitai H, Ishigaki H, Higashiguchi Y, Kondo N, Hirota S, et al. "Tumor-Associated Macrophage-Derived Inflammatory Cytokine Enhances Malignant Potential of Malignant Pleural Mesothelioma." *Cancer Science* 111, no. 8 (August 1, 2020): 2895–2906. https://doi.org/10.1111/CAS.14523.

Jackaman, C, Cornwall S, Graham PT, and Nelson DJ. "CD40-Activated B Cells Contribute to Mesothelioma Tumor Regression." *Immunology and Cell Biology* 89, no. 2 (February 2011): 255–67. https://doi.org/10.1038/ICB.2010.88.

Kennedy, GT, Judy BF, Bhojnagarwala P, Moon EK, Fridlender ZG, Albelda SM, and Singhal S. "Surgical Cytoreduction Restores the Antitumor Efficacy of a Listeria Monocytogenes Vaccine in Malignant

Pleural Mesothelioma." *Immunology Letters* 166, no. 1 (July 1, 2015): 28–35. https://doi.org/10.1016/J.IMLET.2015.05.009.

Klampatsa, A, O'Brien SM, Thompson JC, Rao AS, Stadanlick JE, Martinez MC, Liousia M, et al. "Phenotypic and Functional Analysis of Malignant Mesothelioma Tumor-Infiltrating Lymphocytes." *Oncoimmunology* 8, no. 9 (September 2, 2019). https://doi.org/10.1080/2162402X.2019.1638211.

Kramer, ED, and Abrams SI. "Granulocytic Myeloid-Derived Suppressor Cells as Negative Regulators of Anticancer Immunity." *Frontiers in Immunology* 11 (August 27, 2020). https://doi.org/10.3389/FIMMU.2020.01963.

Kumagai-Takei, N, Lee S, Srinivas B, Shimizu Y, Sada N, Yoshitome K, Ito T, Nishimura Y, and Otsuki T. "The Effects of Asbestos Fibers on Human T Cells." *International Journal of Molecular Sciences* 21, no. 19 (October 1, 2020): 1–13. https://doi.org/10.3390/IJMS21196987.

Kumagai-Takei, N, Nishimura Y, Maeda M, Hayashi H, Matsuzaki H, Lee S, Hiratsuka J, and Otsuki T. "Effect of Asbestos Exposure on Differentiation of Cytotoxic T Lymphocytes in Mixed Lymphocyte Reaction of Human Peripheral Blood Mononuclear Cells." *American Journal of Respiratory Cell and Molecular Biology* 49, no. 1 (July 2013): 28–36. https://doi.org/10.1165/RCMB.2012-0134OC.

Lester, Jason F, Angela C Casbard, Saly Al-Taei, Richard Harrop, Lajos Katona, Richard L Attanoos, Zsuzsanna Tabi, and Gareth O Griffiths. "A Single Centre Phase II Trial to Assess the Immunological Activity of TroVax® plus Pemetrexed/Cisplatin in Patients with Malignant Pleural Mesothelioma – the SKOPOS Trial." *Oncoimmunology* 7, no. 12 (December 2, 2018). https://doi.org/10.1080/2162402X.2018.1457597.

Magkouta, SF, Vaitsi PC, Pappas AG, Iliopoulou M, Kosti CN, Psarra K, and Kalomenidis IT. "CSF1/CSF1R Axis Blockade Limits Mesothelioma and Enhances Efficiency of Anti-PDL1 Immunotherapy." *Cancers* 13, no. 11 (June 1, 2021). https://doi.org/10.3390/CANCERS13112546.

Maio, M, Scherpereel A, Calabrò L, Aerts J, Perez SC, Bearz A, Nackaerts K, et al. "Tremelimumab as Second-Line or Third-Line Treatment in Relapsed Malignant Mesothelioma (DETERMINE): A Multicentre, International, Randomised, Double-Blind, Placebo-Controlled Phase 2b Trial." *The Lancet. Oncology* 18, no. 9 (September 1, 2017): 1261–73. https://doi.org/10.1016/S1470-2045(17)30446-1.

Marabelle, A, Fakih M, Lopez J, Shah M, Shapira-Frommer R, Nakagawa K, Chung HC, et al. "Association of Tumour Mutational Burden with Outcomes in Patients with Advanced Solid Tumours Treated with Pembrolizumab: Prospective Biomarker Analysis of the Multicohort, Open-Label, Phase 2 KEYNOTE-158 Study." *The Lancet. Oncology* 21, no. 10 (October 1, 2020): 1353–65. https://doi.org/10.1016/S1470-2045(20)30445-9.

Marcq, E, Siozopoulou V, De Waele J, van Audenaerde J, Zwaenepoel K, Santermans E, Hens N, Pauwels P, van Meerbeeck JP, and Smits EL. "Prognostic and Predictive Aspects of the Tumor Immune Microenvironment and Immune Checkpoints in Malignant Pleural Mesothelioma." *Oncoimmunology* 6, no. 1 (January 9, 2016). https://doi.org/10.1080/2162402X.2016.1261241.

Marvel, D, and Gabrilovich DI. "Myeloid-Derived Suppressor Cells in the Tumor Microenvironment: Expect the Unexpected." *The Journal of Clinical Investigation* 125, no. 9 (September 1, 2015): 3356–64. https://doi.org/10.1172/JCI80005.

Minnema-Luiting, J, Vroman H, Aerts J, and Cornelissen R. "Heterogeneity in Immune Cell Content in Malignant Pleural Mesothelioma." *International Journal of Molecular Sciences* 19, no. 4 (April 1, 2018). https://doi.org/10.3390/IJMS19041041.

Muller, S, Victoria Lai W, Adusumilli PS, Desmeules P, Frosina D, Jungbluth A, Ni A, et al. "V-Domain Ig-Containing Suppressor of T-Cell Activation (VISTA), a Potentially Targetable Immune Checkpoint Molecule, Is Highly Expressed in Epithelioid Malignant Pleural Mesothelioma." *Modern Pathology : An Official Journal of the United States and Canadian Academy of Pathology, Inc* 33, no. 2 (February 1, 2020): 303–11. https://doi.org/10.1038/S41379-019-0364-Z.

Napoli, F, Listì A, Zambelli V, Witel G, Bironzo P, Papotti M, Volante M, Scagliotti G, and Righi L. "Pathological Characterization of Tumor Immune Microenvironment (TIME) in Malignant Pleural Mesothelioma." *Cancers* 13, no. 11 (June 1, 2021). https://doi.org/10. 3390/CANCERS13112564.

Needham, DJ, Lee JX, and Beilharz MW. "Intra-Tumoural Regulatory T Cells: A Potential New Target in Cancer Immunotherapy." *Biochemical and Biophysical Research Communications* 343, no. 3 (May 12, 2006): 684–91. https://doi.org/10.1016/J.BBRC.2006.03.018.

Neller, MA, López JA, and Schmidt CW. "Antigens for Cancer Immunotherapy." *Seminars in Immunology* 20, no. 5 (October 2008): 286–95. https://doi.org/10.1016/J.SMIM.2008.09.006.

Nowak, AK, Cook AM, McDonnell AM, Millward MJ, Creaney J, Francis RJ, Hasani A, et al. "A Phase 1b Clinical Trial of the CD40-Activating Antibody CP-870,893 in Combination with Cisplatin and Pemetrexed in Malignant Pleural Mesothelioma." *Annals of Oncology : Official Journal of the European Society for Medical Oncology* 26, no. 12 (December 1, 2015): 2483–90. https://doi.org/10.1093/ANNONC/MDV387.

Okada, M, Kijima T, Aoe K, Kato T, Fujimoto N, Nakagawa K, Takeda Y, et al. "Clinical Efficacy and Safety of Nivolumab: Results of a M Ulticenter, Op e n-Label, Single-a r m, Japanese Phase II Study in Mal i Gnant Pleural Meso t Helioma (MERIT)." *Clinical Cancer Research : An Official Journal of the American Association for Cancer Research* 25, no. 18 (September 15, 2019): 5485–92. https://doi.org/10.1158/1078-0432.CCR-19-0103.

Pasello, G, Zago G, Lunardi F, Urso L, Kern I, Vlacic G, Grosso F, et al. "Malignant Pleural Mesothelioma Immune Microenvironment and Checkpoint Expression: Correlation with Clinical-Pathological Features and Intratumor Heterogeneity over Time." *Annals of Oncology : Official Journal of the European Society for Medical Oncology* 29, no. 5 (May 1, 2018): 1258–65. https://doi.org/10.1093/ANNONC/MDY086.

Patil, NS, Righi L, Koeppen H, Zou W, Izzo S, Grosso F, Libener R, et al. "Molecular and Histopathological Characterization of the Tumor Immune Microenvironment in Advanced Stage of Malignant Pleural Mesothelioma." *Journal of Thoracic Oncology : Official Publication of the International Association for the Study of Lung Cancer* 13, no. 1 (January 1, 2018): 124–33. https://doi.org/10.1016/J.JTHO.2017.09.1968.

Petrausch, U, Schuberth PC, Hagedorn C, Soltermann A, Tomaszek S, Stahel R, Weder W, and Renner C. "Re-Directed T Cells for the Treatment of Fibroblast Activation Protein (FAP)-Positive Malignant Pleural Mesothelioma (FAPME-1)." *BMC Cancer* 12 (December 22, 2012). https://doi.org/10.1186/1471-2407-12-615.

Pezzuto, F, Lunardi F, Vedovelli L, Fortarezza F, Urso L, Grosso F, Ceresoli GL, et al. "P14/ARF-Positive Malignant Pleural Mesothelioma: A Phenotype With Distinct Immune Microenvironment." *Frontiers in Oncology* 11 (March 22, 2021). https://doi.org/10.3389/FONC.2021.653497.

Popat, S, Curioni-Fontecedro A, Dafni U, Shah R, O'Brien M, Pope A, Fisher P, et al. "A Multicentre Randomised Phase III Trial Comparing Pembrolizumab versus Single-Agent Chemotherapy for Advanced Pre-Treated Malignant Pleural Mesothelioma: The European Thoracic Oncology Platform (ETOP 9-15) PROMISE-Meso Trial." *Annals of Oncology : Official Journal of the European Society for Medical Oncology* 31, no. 12 (December 1, 2020): 1734–45. https://doi.org/10.1016/J.ANNONC.2020.09.009.

Powell, A, Creaney J, Broomfield S, Van Bruggen I, and Robinson B. "Recombinant GM-CSF plus Autologous Tumor Cells as a Vaccine for Patients with Mesothelioma." *Lung Cancer (Amsterdam, Netherlands)* 52, no. 2 (May 2006): 189–97. https://doi.org/10.1016/J.LUNGCAN.2006.01.007.

Powell, Alex, Jenette Creaney, Steven Broomfield, Ivonne Van Bruggen, and Bruce Robinson. "Recombinant GM-CSF plus Autologous Tumor Cells as a Vaccine for Patients with Mesothelioma." *Lung Cancer* 52, no. 2 (May 1, 2006): 189–97. https://doi.org/10.1016/J.LUNGCAN. 2006.01.007.

Quispel-Janssen, J, van der Noort V, de Vries JF, Zimmerman M, Lalezari F, Thunnissen E, Monkhorst K, et al. "Programmed Death 1 Blockade With Nivolumab in Patients With Recurrent Malignant Pleural Mesothelioma." *Journal of Thoracic Oncology : Official Publication of the International Association for the Study of Lung Cancer* 13, no. 10 (October 1, 2018): 1569–76. https://doi.org/10.1016/J.JTHO.2018. 05.038.

Robinson, Bruce WS, Arthur W Musk, and Richard A Lake. "Malignant Mesothelioma." *The Lancet* 366, no. 9483 (July 30, 2005): 397–408. https://doi.org/10.1016/S0140-6736(05)67025-0.

Robinson, BW, Mukherjee SA, Davidson A, Morey S, Musk AW, Ramshaw I, Smith D, et al. "Cytokine Gene Therapy or Infusion as Treatment for Solid Human Cancer." *Journal of Immunotherapy* (Hagerstown, Md. : 1997) 21, no. 3 (1998): 211–17. https://doi.org/10. 1097/00002371-199805000-00007.

Robinson, BW, Robinson C, and Lake RA. "Localised Spontaneous Regression in Mesothelioma -- Possible Immunological Mechanism." *Lung Cancer (Amsterdam, Netherlands)* 32, no. 2 (2001): 197–201. https://doi.org/10.1016/S0169-5002(00)00217-8.

Robinson, C, Callow M, Stevenson S, Scott B, Robinson BW, and Lake RA. "Serologic Responses in Patients with Malignant Mesothelioma: Evidence for Both Public and Private Specificities." *American Journal of Respiratory Cell and Molecular Biology* 22, no. 5 (2000): 550–56. https://doi.org/10.1165/AJRCMB.22.5.3930.

Sahin, U, and Türeci Ö. "Personalized Vaccines for Cancer Immunotherapy." *Science (New York, N.Y.)* 359, no. 6382 (March 1, 2018): 1355–60. https://doi.org/10.1126/SCIENCE.AAR7112.

Sakaguchi, S, Yamaguchi T, Nomura T, and Ono M. "Regulatory T Cells and Immune Tolerance." *Cell* 133, no. 5 (May 30, 2008): 775–87. https://doi.org/10.1016/J.CELL.2008.05.009.

Salaroglio, IC, Kopecka J, Napoli F, Pradotto M, Maletta F, Costardi L, Gagliasso M, et al. "Potential Diagnostic and Prognostic Role of

Microenvironment in Malignant Pleural Mesothelioma." *Journal of Thoracic Oncology : Official Publication of the International Association for the Study of Lung Cancer* 14, no. 8 (August 1, 2019): 1458–71. https://doi.org/10.1016/J.JTHO.2019.03.029.

Scherpereel, A, Mazieres J, Greillier L, Lantuejoul S, Dô P, Bylicki O, Monnet I, et al. "Nivolumab or Nivolumab plus Ipilimumab in Patients with Relapsed Malignant Pleural Mesothelioma (IFCT-1501 MAPS2): A Multicentre, Open-Label, Randomised, Non-Comparative, Phase 2 Trial." *The Lancet. Oncology* 20, no. 2 (February 1, 2019): 239–53. https://doi.org/10.1016/S1470-2045(18)30765-4.

Sekido. Y, "Molecular Pathogenesis of Malignant Mesothelioma." *Carcinogenesis* 34, no. 7 (July 2013): 1413–19. https://doi.org/10.1093/CARCIN/BGT166.

Serke, Monika, and R Loddenkemper. "Therapeutische Optionen Beim Malignen Pleuramesotheliom." *Pneumologie* 59, no. 5 (May 2005): 337–48.

Srivastava, Shivani, and Stanley R Riddell. "CAR T Cell Therapy: Challenges to Bench-to-Bedside Efficacy." *Journal of Immunology (Baltimore, Md. : 1950)* 200, no. 2 (January 15, 2018): 459. https://doi.org/10.4049/JIMMUNOL.1701155.

Thapa, B, M Walkeiwicz, G Rivalland, C Murone, K Asadi, S Barnett, S Knight, S Hendry, P Russell, and T John. "OA08.05 Quantifying Tumour Infiltrating Lymphocytes (TILs) in Malignant Pleural Mesothelioma (MPM) -Defining the Hot, the Warm and the Cold Tumours." *Journal of Thoracic Oncology* 13, no. 10 (October 1, 2018): S339. https://doi.org/10.1016/J.JTHO.2018.08.278.

Toh, B, Wang X, Keeble J, Sim WJ, Khoo K, Wong WC, Kato M, Prevost-Blondel A, Thiery JP, and Abastado JP. "Mesenchymal Transition and Dissemination of Cancer Cells Is Driven by Myeloid-Derived Suppressor Cells Infiltrating the Primary Tumor." *PLoS Biology* 9, no. 9 (September 2011). https://doi.org/10.1371/JOURNAL.PBIO.1001162.

Upham, JW, Musk AW, van Hazel G, Byrne M, and Robinson BW. "Interferon Alpha and Doxorubicin in Malignant Mesothelioma: A

Phase II Study." *Australian and New Zealand Journal of Medicine* 23, no. 6 (1993): 683–87. https://doi.org/10.1111/J.1445-5994.1993.TB04727.X.

Wagner, JC, Sleggs CA, and Marchand P. "Diffuse Pleural Mesothelioma and Asbestos Exposure in the North Western Cape Province." *British Journal of Industrial Medicine* 17, no. 4 (October 1, 1960): 260–71. https://doi.org/10.1136/OEM.17.4.260.

Xia, Y, Xie Y, Yu Z, Xiao H, Jiang G, Zhou X, Yang Y, et al. "The Mevalonate Pathway Is a Druggable Target for Vaccine Adjuvant Discovery." *Cell* 175, no. 4 (November 1, 2018): 1059-1073.e21. https://doi.org/10.1016/J.CELL.2018.08.070.

Yap, TA, Aerts JG, Popat S, and Fennell DA. "Novel Insights into Mesothelioma Biology and Implications for Therapy." *Nature Reviews. Cancer* 17, no. 8 (July 25, 2017): 475–88. https://doi.org/10.1038/NRC.2017.42.

Zalcman, Gerard, Solange Peters, Aaron Scott Mansfield, Thierry Marie Jahan, Sanjay Popat, Arnaud Scherpereel, Wenhua Hu, Giovanni Selvaggi, and Paul Baas. *"Checkmate 743: A Phase 3, Randomized, Open-Label Trial of Nivolumab (Nivo) plus Ipilimumab (Ipi) vs Pemetrexed plus Cisplatin or Carboplatin as First-Line Therapy in Unresectable Pleural Mesothelioma."* Https://Doi.Org/10.1200/JCO.2017.35.15_suppl.TPS8581 35, no. 15_suppl (May 30, 2017): TPS8581–TPS8581. https://doi.org/10.1200/JCO.2017.35.15_SUPPL.TPS8581.

Zauderer, MG, Tsao AS, Dao T, Panageas K, Lai WV, Rimner A, Rusch VW, et al. "A Randomized Phase II Trial of Adjuvant Galinpepimut-S, WT-1 Analogue Peptide Vaccine, After Multimodality Therapy for Patients with Malignant Pleural Mesothelioma." *Clinical Cancer Research : An Official Journal of the American Association for Cancer Research* 23, no. 24 (2017): 7483–89. https://doi.org/10.1158/1078-0432.CCR-17-2169.

Zhou, J, Tang Z, Gao S, Li C, Feng Y, and Zhou X. "Tumor-Associated Macrophages: Recent Insights and Therapies." *Frontiers in Oncology* 10 (February 25, 2020). https://doi.org/10.3389/FONC.2020.00188.

Zhu, Y, Knolhoff BL, Meyer MA, Nywening TM, West BL, Luo J, Wang-Gillam A, Goedegebuure SP, Linehan DC, and DeNardo DG. "CSF1/CSF1R Blockade Reprograms Tumor-Infiltrating Macrophages and Improves Response to T-Cell Checkpoint Immunotherapy in Pancreatic Cancer Models." *Cancer Research* 74, no. 18 (July 31, 2014): 5057–69. https://doi.org/10.1158/0008-5472.CAN-13-3723.

In: Mesothelioma
Editor: Albert K. Martin

ISBN: 978-1-68507-075-5
© 2021 Nova Science Publishers, Inc.

Chapter 2

MALIGNANT MESOTHELIOMA

Anwar M. Alesawi[*], *Faisal S. Mandourah and Hasan M. Alesawi*
Fakeeh Care, Jeddah, Saudi Arabia

ABSTRACT

Malignant Mesothelioma (MM) is an insidious neoplasm arising from mesothelial surfaces i.e., pleura (65%-70%), peritoneum (30%), tunica vaginalis testis, and pericardium (1%-2%). It is a rare but rapidly fatal and aggressive tumor with limited knowledge of its natural history. The earliest mention of a possible tumor of the chest wall (the pleura) was made in 1767 by Joseph Lieutaud, while Peritoneal mesothelioma was first described in 1908 by Miller and Wynn. The incidence is approximately 2500 per year in the United States. Comparing to lung cancer, incidence is more than 160,000 new cases per year. Asbestos exposure plays a critical role in malignant pleural mesothelioma in the United States. There are several risk factors that linked to development of malignant mesothelioma like ionizing radiation, genetic susceptibility,

---

[*] Corresponding Author's E-mail: esawi_anwar@yahoo.com.

exposure to particular viruses like simian virus 40, but still occupational and environmental asbestos exposure remains a major causative factor.

Treatment of malignant mesothelioma range from surgery to radiation and chemotherapy, but preventive measures like taking the appropriate precautions if you are exposed to asbestos at work is a major part of management.

INTRODUCTION

Malignant Mesothelioma (MM) is a rare but rapidly fatal and aggressive tumor of the pleura and peritoneum with limited knowledge of its natural history. The earliest mention of the chest wall (the pleura) possible tumor was made in 1767 by Joseph Lieutaud, the founder of pathologic anatomy in France in study of 3,000 autopsies, where two cases of "pleural tumors" were found. In 1819, René-Théophile-Hyacinthe Laennec, the French physician, suggested the origin from the pleura based upon his understanding of the nature of pleural cells.

Peritoneal mesothelioma was first described in 1908 by Miller and Wynn [1]. The disease incidence varies geographically (i.e., from less than 1 per 1,000,000 in Tunisia and Morocco, to the highest rate in Britain, Australia and Belgium i.e., 30 per 1,000,000 per year) [2]. Currently, the incidence ranges from about 7 to 40 per 1,000,000 in industrialized Western nations, depending upon the amount of asbestos exposure in the past several decades [3].

Mesothelioma is an insidious neoplasm arising from mesothelium. i.e., pleura (65%-70%), peritoneum (30%), tunica Vaginalis testis, and pericardium (1%-2%) [1.]

The overall prevalence in the United States is 1-2 cases per million or 3300 cases every year from which only 10 to 15 percent (200 -400 new cases annually) are peritoneal mesothelioma, [4] the incidence rates of Malignant Peritoneal Mesothelioma have remained stable over the last 30 years though [5, 6].

On the other hand, primary malignant mesothelioma is a highly aggressive malignancy that occurs most commonly in older men and has a real and strong association with high levels of occupational asbestos exposure [7, 8]. It occur more common in male than female, as the incidence of peritoneal mesothelioma is 0.5–3.0 per million per year in male, and 0.2–2.0 per million per year in female [9]. The female component was particularly lower for extra peritoneal MM, with male/female ratios of 1.4:1 and 1.9:1 for peritoneal and pericardium, respectively, compared to 2.7 male pleural MM cases for each female [10].

It can occur in any age group but more prevalent in 6th decade and only about 2% to 5% of all cases reported in the first two decades of life [10].

RISK FACTORS

Frequent asbestos inhalation predisposes to malignant pleural mesothelioma subsequent to repeated pleural inflammation, production of hazardous free radical, oncogenic activation, and interference with mitosis. This mesothelioma may be associated with ionizing radiation and a germline mutation of BRCA 1 Associated Protein (BAP1). However, neither alcohol nor smoking are linked with malignant pleural mesothelioma, despite the significantly increased risk of lung cancer with smoking [11].

Asbestos

Occupational and environmental asbestos exposure remains a major causative factor, including amosite and crocidolite. It is more common in male than female and can appear at any age in either sex but the risk increases with age. Incidence of Malignant Peritoneal Mesothelioma (MPM) is less when compared to pleural mesothelioma, it is 20% to 33% of all mesotheliomas, one fifth to one third of (MM) arises from the peritoneum [12].

All forms of mesothelioma are strongly associated with industrial pollutants, of which asbestos is the principal carcinogen. Among Asbestos (primarily the crocidolite variety) is considered the main risk factor. Other risk factors in some patients are radiation exposure, talc, erionite (*Erionite is a potent carcinogenic mineral fiber capable of causing both pleural and peritoneal MM.*) or mica exposure, and patients suffering from familial Mediterranean fever and diffuse lymphocytic lymphoma. Literature review shows that only 50% of patients with a peritoneal origin of MPM have a history of asbestos exposure [12, 6]. Most researchers reported that the possible point of origin for MM is the membrane where the cancer develops from, is composed of mesothelial cells, which are present in most of the body's membranous linings.

Asbestos can induces DNA alterations, mostly by inducing mesothelial cells and reactive macrophages to secrete mutagenic nitrogen species and oxygen. In addition, asbestos carcinogenesis is linked to the chronic inflammatory process caused by the deposition of a sufficient number of asbestos fibers and the consequent release of pro-inflammatory molecules, especially TNF-alpha and HMGB-1, the master switch that starts the inflammatory process by mesothelial cells and macrophages.

Carbone et al, reported that radiation exposure, genetic predisposition and viral infection are co-factors that can together with asbestos and erionite or alone cause MM [13].

While there is currently no theory to explain how asbestos exposure might cause mesothelial cells to develop primary tumor, it is understood that once the asbestos fibers enter the body, they lodge in organs and cause infection or inflammation. Eventually, this can result in the development of mesothelioma. These fibers potentiate cancerous cells to divide abnormally, causing buildup of fluid and formation of tumors [13].

People Most at Risk of an Asbestos-Related Disease

Workplaces were once a common place for some workers to be exposed to asbestos.

Occupations that carried the most risk of being exposed to asbestos are:

- Miners
- Shipyard workers
- Ceramics industry workers
- Cement manufacturer with asbestos
- Automotive workers, especially those who manufactured break linings and clutches
- Railroad Workers
- Insulation Manufacturers And Installers
- Construction workers
- Gas mask manufacturers
- Firefighters demolition workers [14].

Non-Occupational Exposure

1) Ionizing radiation: Therapeutic or nontherapeutic ionizing radiation to the human body may be a risk factor for the subsequent development of MM, with a long latent period [15, 16].
2) Exposure to a particular: Oncogenic viral infections, such as Simian virus 40 infections, have a role in the etiology of malignant peritoneal mesothelioma (MPM) [17, 18], although a clear relationship has yet to be identified [19, 20].
3) Genetic susceptibility: Inactivation of the nuclear deubiquitinase BRCA1-associated protein 1 (BAP1), an important regulator of transcription factors related to tumorgenesis, has been associated with MM [21, 22]. Germ line mutations in *BAP1* were identified in two families with high incidence of MM [23] and *BAP1* inactivation through somatic mutations was detected in 23% of MM tumor tissues [24].

These emerging data suggest that individuals with loss of BAP1 may have higher MM development risk, mainly after asbestos exposure. Close monitoring and early intervention might be warranted, although genetic screening strategies have yet to be established [25].

It is believed that particular genetic makeup or changes may make people more susceptible to this disease. Research shows that the loss of one copy of chromosome 22 is commonly seen in patients with malignant pleural mesothelioma. Other chromosomal anomalies that have been identified include deletions in chromosomal arms 3p, 1p, 6q, and 9p.

Histopathology and Pathophysiology

Malignant pleural mesothelioma has three histological subtypes, including sarcomatous, mixed, and epithelial variants, where the epithelium type has the best prognosis. Excised tissue usually reveals multifocal large nodules on the pleural, starting at the parietal pleura. Local extension to the visceral pleura precedes spread to the chest wall, diaphragm, and mediastinum. The pattern of nodal metastases is different from that seen in lung cancer, where local lymph nodes are directly invaded. Although nodal involvement in malignant pleural mesothelioma is not common, bronchopulmonary and hilar lymph nodes are primarily affected before the carinal, internal mammary or peri-diaphragmatic nodes.

Presentation

Chest pain and dyspnea represents the most commonly presenting symptoms of malignant pleural mesothelioma. Dyspnea mostly suggests the presence of pleural effusion, which is commonly detected at initial examination in about 90% of patients. Non-specific symptoms may be reported such as loss of appetite, unintentional weight loss, cough, fatigue, and chest wall mass.

Evaluation

Malignant pleural mesothelioma should be differentiated from other entities such as benign pleural diseases and secondary metastasis of other tumors, including lung adenocarcinoma or chest wall sarcoma. Initial workup includes an enhanced chest CT scan, a thoracoscopic pleural biopsy, and thoracentesis of pleural effusion, if present, with cytologic analysis. A chest CT scan may show focal areas of pleural thickening, with a large invasive mass in late-stage of the disease. PET scans may be used to screen for metastatic disease, while MRI and laparoscopy can be used to evaluate diaphragmatic invasion. Megakaryocyte potentiating factor is a serum biomarker for diagnosis of malignant pleural mesothelioma. A stress electrocardiography should be performed and pulmonary function tests should be optimized in all patients before surgery.

TREATMENT

The diagnosis of mesothelioma (MM) is often delayed, as a result of the long latent period between onset and symptoms and the nonspecific clinical presentation.

Due to its unusual nature, this disease has not been clearly defined in terms of its natural history, diagnosis or management. Moreover, the treatment options available are far from satisfactory. As an example, malignant peritoneal mesothelioma (MPM) usually remains confined to the peritoneal cavity during most of its natural history, so cytoreductive regional chemotherapy is an attractive option in management [26].

Because of this lack of effective treatment, median survival time is 5 to 12 months, and mean symptoms-to-survival time is one year [27, 28].

The National Comprehensive Cancer Network (NCCN) Guidelines, treatment recommended appropriate tumor staging to assess the feasibility of surgical resection. Stage III-IV malignant pleural mesothelioma are considered unresectable. In addition, mesothelioma should be treated by a multidisciplinary team at a high volume center, with less than one third of patients are candidates for definitive resection [29].

Preventive Measures

The most important thing to prevent mesothelioma is by using appropriate precautions if you are exposed to asbestos at work.

Occupational safety and health administration (OSHA) has asbestos safety *standards* for individuals who may be exposed at work.

It is important for all workers with asbestos, to follow these guidelines to minimize their families' exposure as well. Asbestos insulation in homes is often not a problem, unless it is damaged or disturbed by projects of remodeling. Those people with asbestos insulation at home (homes built prior to 1950) should make sure to hire a contractor certified in asbestos management before they begin any improvement projects at home.

People exposed to asbestos should consider work up like CT screening. Recommendations for screening include those people aged 55 to 74 with a 30 year history of smoking.

Curative Measures

Surgical

Depends on the stage of Mesothelioma and is divided into 2 primary stages:

- Localized (Stage I) – With localized mesothelioma, the cancer is confined to the origin like pleura, pericardium, peritoneum and tunica vaginalis.
- Advanced (Stage II, III, and IV) – Mesothelioma is considered advanced if it has spread to the surrounding organs or tissues, lymph nodes, or other distant organs.

Malignant Mesothelioma of Tunica Vaginalis

Malignant mesothelioma of the tunica vaginalis of the testis is a rare entity representing less than 1% of all mesothelioma. It may be initially misdiagnosed as a hydrocele or an epididymal cyst. An aggressive approach with hemiscrotectomy with or without inguinal and retroperitoneal lymphadenectomy can reduce the risk of recurrence. Surgery is the only curative treatment for MM of tunica vaginalis. Radical inguinal orchidectomy and hemiscrotectomy is the standard recommended treatment. Lymph node dissection is controversial. Despite this form of mesothelioma being much localized it is still associated with poor outcome, only 5% of patients survive beyond 5 years. There is no evidence to support radiotherapy and chemotherapy in the treatment of the disease [30]. Adjuvant radiotherapy could be considered in locally advanced or metastatic disease [31].

The mean disease-specific survival for patients with or without systemic treatment was 26 and 36 months, respectively [32]. Given the rarity of mesothelioma of the testicle, the best treatment is difficult to precise.

We (Alesawi et al. [33]) reported a case of rare malignant mesothelioma of the tunica Vaginalis with no history of exposure to asbestos with a comprehensive literature review. The diagnosis of malignant mesothelioma of tunica Vaginalis testis is sometimes missed in case of the absence of nodules on physical examination or scrotal ultrasound scan. Histopathological examination with immunohistochemistry is considered the way of confirming the diagnosis of MM of tunica vaginalis.

Malignant Pleural Mesothelioma

Surgery is used for staging procedures or with palliative or curative intent. In MPM using video assisted thoracic surgery (VATS) or thoracoscopy, large biopsy samples can be obtained for proper pathological, molecular analyses. During this procedure, the local extent of the tumour can be examined. Pleural effusions can be drained and, if required, a pleurodesis or decortication can be carried out. Surgery for staging involves the extension of the tumour on the pleural lining and invasion of muscle layers, while thoracoscopic inspection of the pleural cavity can be used in some cases. Besides this intervention, the staging procedure can also be used to control pleural effusion, and to perform a talc poudrage or even decortication in cases of a captured lung. One study compared VATS (partial) pleurectomy versus standard talc poudrage in 196 patients [34].

The IASLC (International association for the study of lung cancer) established a working group to recommend uniform definitions for surgical procedures dealing with mesothelioma [35]. Currently, a clear distinction is made between EPP (Extra pleural pneumonectomy) and pleurectomy/decortication (P/D) with different subcategories: EPP implies an en bloc complete removal of the involved parietal and visceral pleura including the whole ipsilateral lung. If required, the pericardium and diaphragm can also be resected. In a retrospective analysis of data from three large institutions, 663 patients who underwent an EPP or P/D were examined for survival outcome and toxicity [36]. The operative mortality was slightly higher (7%) for EPP compared with P/D (4%), with a higher OS of 16 months for P/D versus 12 months for EPP. Different combined modality regimens have been investigated including some studies that reported about a trimodality approach in order to obtain cure. In locally advanced lung cancer, induction chemotherapy was considered to increase the complete resection rate of early- stage mesothelioma. A Swiss multicentre trial reported on their experience with additive effect of radiation therapy after a combination of three cycles of cisplatin and gemcitabine as induction therapy followed by EPP in patients with resectable MM [37]. Complete resection was obtained in 37/61 (61%) patients and 36 patients received postoperative RT. The 90-day mortality was 3.2%.

Radical resection is the preferred treatment in malignant peritoneal mesotheliomais and is associated with a better prognoses and should be pursued when possible [38, 39].

Other treatments consist of intensive loco-regional therapeutic strategies such as cytoreductive surgery, hyperthermic intraoperative or early postoperative intraperitoneal chemotherapy and immunotherapy.

Radical resection is often not possible, so, the better option is to perform cytoreductive surgery which is aimed to remove as much tumor as possible [40]. The surgical debulking is classified according to the Completeness of Cytoreduction Score which is also widely used in both invasive and noninvasive malignancies. This is defined as the evaluation of residual peritoneal seeding within the operative field and is thought to be the principle prognostic indicator. Completeness of Cytoreduction Score comprises of complete cytoreduction (CC-0) or partial with a diameter of the residual nodules < 0.25 cm (CC-1), 0.25-2.5 cm (CC-2) and > 2.5 cm or confluence of tumor nodules (CC-3) [39, 40].

The CC-1 tumor is considered penetrable by intracavitary chemotherapy and is, therefore, designated as complete cytoreduction if perioperative intraperitoneal chemotherapy is used. This can be evaluated only after surgery therefore; no preoperative assessment about resectability of the tumor can be done which is considered as a limitation to this scoring system [43]. Mean Survival after cytoreductive surgery and intraperitoneal chemotherapy is 35.8 months in CC-0 or CC-1 resection, and only 6.5 months with a CC-2 or CC-3 resection [45].

CHEMOTHERAPY

Malignant pleural mesothelioma is more resistant to chemotherapy with unclear survival benefits. However, platinum-based chemotherapeutic agents such as cisplatin are the first treatment option for unresectable disease. Combined gemcitabine and cisplatin have a response rate of 12-48%, with a median overall survival of only 9-13 months. Currently, biologic and antiangiogenic therapies are being investigated. Intraperitoneally or systemically has an important role in palliative treatment. Moreover, direct exposure of antitumor agent to the peritoneal surface is considered to be most effective against malignant peritoneal mesothelioma. Literature review shows that the overall response rate with a single agent, combined, intraperitoneal chemotherapy and continuous hyperthermic peritoneal perfusion are 13.1%, 20.5%, 47.4%, and 84.6%, respectively [44].

Intraperitoneal chemotherapy can be instilled after surgery or without surgery through an abdominal catheter. Intraperitoneal chemotherapy advantages include less systemic toxicity and greatly enhanced drug concentrations in the peritoneal cavity [45].

Several studies reported that continuous intraperitoneal hyperthermic perfusion after cytoreductive surgery for resectable tumors is the standard treatment at diagnosis [40, 46, 47]. Preheated (42.5 degrees C) perfusate with 2 or 3 antineoplastic agents (i.e., Cisplatin, Mitomycin C, Fluorouracil, Doxorubicin, and/or Paclitaxel) is continuously infused after surgery into the closed or semi-closed abdomen. Up to 12% of major morbidities are reported in literature and the most significant complications are anastomotic leaks (11%), abdominal bleeds (1.9%) and sepsis (1.9%) [38, 45].

About 12% operative mortality is also reported. Cisplatin was the most studied chemotherapeutic agent, with activity in 25% of patients [48].

Literature shows that the Pemetrexed in combination with cisplatin has improved survival in patients with peritoneal mesothelioma as in pleural mesothelioma when they are used as systemic chemotherapy [49, 50]. Data recommends it as a standard of care for patients with unresectable MM. These data reported about 71.2% of the disease control rate that includes partial responses or stable disease. Complete responses where not reported with this chemotherapy [51].

Other regimens like Vinorelbine and Gemcitabine, either alone or combined with platinum compounds where also used for unresectable disease [50]. The response rate of Vinorelbine alone was 24% [51]. Whereas the Irinotecan and Gefinitib have not proved effective when used alone. 50,51 Overall survival of 70%, with 63%, disease-free survival, and 51% progression-free survival after cytoreductive surgery and continuous hyperthermic peritoneal perfusion with Cisplatin, Fluorouracil, and Paclitaxel reported in literature [46].

Over the past two decades, the management of peritoneal mesothelioma has evolved similarly to ovarian cancer treatment i.e., cytoreductive surgery, heated intraoperative intraperitoneal chemotherapy (HIIC) with cisplatin, doxorubicin, and early postoperative intraperitoneal paclitaxel. These perioperative treatments are followed by adjuvant intraperitoneal Paclitaxel and second-look cytoreduction. This multimodality treatment has resulted in a median survival of 50 to 60 months [54, 56].

RADIOTHERAPY

Radiation therapy is used in M.M by utilizing high-energy x-rays or other types of radiation to kill cancer cells or keep them from growing. There are two types of radiation therapy:

- External radiation therapy: uses a machine outside the body to send radiation toward cancers.
- Internal radiation therapy: uses a radioactive substance sealed in needles, seeds, wires, or catheters that are placed directly into or near the cancer.

The way the radiation therapy is given depends on the type and stage of the cancer being treated.

Radiotherapy (RT) can be used for different indications in mesothelioma: as a preventive management, as palliation and as part of a multimodality treatment. However, the results are extremely poor. The treatment does not affect survival but may provide palliation in patients with chest wall metastasis.

For patients suffering from pain due to bone involvement, short course regimens of RT (such as 1×10 or 3×8 Gy), usually can be considered although the systematic review by Macleod et al. [56, 57] reported that no high-quality evidence currently exists to support RT in treating pain in MM. In the case of palliation.

There is much debate whether a scar after thoracoscopy and/or drainage procedures should be irradiated as a prophylaxis in order to reduce the likelihood of metastases by seeding. It might be better to recommend refraining from this procedure unless in the setting of a clinical trial [58] such as the United Kingdom 'PIT' study (ClinicalTrials.gov Identifier NCT01604005). A randomised trial compared immediate drain site RT (21 Gy in three fractions) to observation in 61 patients treated between 1998 and 2004 [57]. The authors concluded that prophylactic drain site RT in MPM did not decrease the incidence of seeding metastasis, as indicated by previous studies conducted in the 1990s. Quality control of RT, the use of first-line therapy and patient selection can probably explain the discrepancy of these results.

Generally, it is not recommended that RT is administered before or after surgery with large fields (hemi-thoracic RT). The results are poor, in terms of local control, because of the complex growth patterns in the diaphragm gutters and in the lobar fissures. The field size and neighbouring vital organs contribute considerably to toxicity.

Radiation-induced lung toxicity is high, especially when the lung remains in situ after decortication. 3D planning and the introduction of intensity- modulated RT (IMRT) improved most of these issues and allow the remaining tumour tissue to be properly irradiated. The 'SMART' study is investigating a short accelerated course of high-dose hemithoracic IMRT followed by extra pleural pneumonectomy (EPP) [60].

In the absence of phase III randomised trials, the establishment of a prospective controlled study evaluating the efficacy and tolerability of adjuvant RT post-EPP is recommended. In this study, a minimum recommended dose of 50 Gy, with a daily fraction size of 1.8–2 Gy should be given. In one study, hemithoracic irradiation (54 Gy) was given as adjuvant therapy after EPP [61]. The local recurrence rate was 13%, with a 4% local- only recurrence rate.

Preliminary results of IMRT in the adjuvant setting after EPP seemed particularly promising. IMRT may provide good local control with protection of at risk organs such as the heart or liver. Even after removal of one entire lung, fatal pulmonary toxicity remained a problem, with six out of 13 patients developing fatal pneumonitis [62]. Further studies are needed to better establish the role of RT. Recent studies have underlined the importance of RT technique, both in terms of local control and toxicity. It is therefore recommended that RT should be delivered in specialized centers (expert advice).

Recommendation

Radiation therapy can be considered in the following cases:

- For palliation of pain related to tumor growth, RT can be considered [II, A].
- The use of RT to prevent growth in drainage tracts is not proved to be useful [III, A].
- RT can be given in an adjuvant setting after surgery or chemo-surgery to reduce the local recurrence rate. However, no evidence is available for its use as a standard treatment [II, A].
- When postoperative RT is applied, strict constraints must be adhered to in order to avoid toxicity to neighbouring organs, and special tissue sparing, techniques should be used [II, A].

TARGETED THERAPY

The need for more effective therapies for MM has prompted basic research to identify novel therapeutic targets. For example, epigenetic regulation of tumor suppressor genes has emerged as an important mechanism that leads to tumor development and growth. Inhibition of DNA transcription by the histone deacetylase family proteins (HDACs), through histone modifications, and its overexpression and/or aberrant function have been found in mesothelioma as well as many other cancers [63, 64].

Vorinostat is one of the best-studied HDAC inhibitors and currently is approved by the U.S. Food and Drug Administration for cutaneous T-cell lymphoma treatment. The original phase I trial of vorinostat included 13 patients with MPM, and 2 of them had a partial response (15.4%) [65]. This has led to a multicenter phase III study (VANTAGE 014) of vorinostat in patients who progressed after first-line chemotherapy. This large randomized trial in mesothelioma (660 patients) has failed to show a benefit in OS (30.7 versus 27.1 weeks, $p = 0.858$) and only a marginal improvement in PFS (6.3 versus 6.1 weeks, $p < 0.001$) [64].

Mesothelioma cells release and express several angiogenic factors such as platelet-derived growth factor (PDGF), PDGF receptor (PDGFR), vascular endothelial growth factor (VEGF), VEGF receptor (VEGFR), and fibroblast growth factor receptor (FGFR) [65]. Bevacizumab, an anti-VEGF monoclonal antibody, did not significantly improve either PFS or OS in patients with advanced MM when it was added to first-line gemcitabine-cisplatin chemotherapy [68].

Bevacizumab was evaluated in another phase II trial in addition to first- line pemetrexed and cisplatin but failed to achieve its primary endpoint (33% improvement in PFS at 6 months compared with historical controls) [69].

Interim analysis from a French multicenteric randomized phase II/III trial of pemetrexed and cisplatin with or without bevacizumab (MAPS) was recently reported [70]. Compared to chemotherapy alone. Patients in the bevacizumab arm had a RR of 14% and a better disease control (73.5% versus 43.2%; $p = .01$) at 6 months. This trial will hopefully complete recruitment soon [69], and its final results are expected to clarify the role of bevacizumab in MM management.

Nintedanib is a potent oral triple angiokinase inhibitor that targets all three major angiogenic pathways [72]. It showed an acceptable safety profile and antitumor activities in phase I/II clinical trials [73]. Second-line nintedanib plus docetaxel, in the phase III LUME-Lung 1 study for patients with non- small cell lung cancer, significantly improved PFS compared with docetaxel alone (3.4 versus 2.7 months; $p = .0019$) and improved OS in patients with adenocarcinoma histology (12.6 versus 10.3 months; $p = .0359$) [72].

Nintedanib in combination with pemetrexed and cisplatin followed by maintenance nintedanib compared with chemotherapy alone in patients with unresectable MM will be evaluated in an ongoing randomized multicenter phase II trial. SWOG is also studying the addition of the oral anti-VEGFR tyrosine kinase inhibitor cediranib versus placebo to pemetrexed-cisplatin in a randomized phase II trial.

Activation of multiple mitogenic signaling pathways, including focal adhesion kinase (FAK) pathways and the mammalian target of rapamycin (mTOR) can be caused by the loss of the tumor suppressor protein moesin-ezrin-radixin-like protein (merlin) [75]. About 40% of MM patients carry inactivating mutations in the neurofibromin 2 (*NF2*) gene, which encodes for merlin [76, 77], and overexpression of FAK has been implicated in increased invasiveness of mesothelioma [76].

Merlin loss may result in improved PFS response to FAK inhibition. This was suggested by a recently reported phase I study of GSK2256098 (an oral FAK inhibitor; GlaxoSmithKline, Brentford, U.K., http://www.gsk.com) that included 23 patients with recurrent MM [79].

A phase II randomized multicenter study of defactinib maintenance (VS- 6063; Verastem, Cambridge, MA, http://www.verastem.com) is a highly potent, selective FAK inhibitor) in MPM patients who have not progressed after first-line pemetrexed-platinum chemotherapy is actively recruiting.

The phosphatidylinositol 3-kinase (PI3K), AKT, and mTOR (PI3K/AKT/mTOR) pathway is one of the key regulators in cell survival, proliferation, and apoptosis [80]. Aberrant signaling cascade has been demonstrated in several cancer types, including MM [81, 82]. Merlin and mTOR loss has become a target of interest in MM because merlin is a negative regulator of the mTOR pathway [83]. The mTOR inhibitor rapamycin showed a much enhanced growth-inhibitory effect on merlin-negative mesothelioma cells compared with merlin-positive cells [84].

A SWOG phase II study of post-front-line mTOR inhibitor everolimus (RAD001) failed to show activity in unselected patients [83]. GDC-0980 (Genentech, South San Francisco, CA, http://www.gene.com) is a potent, selective oral PI3K/mTOR dual inhibitor that has demonstrated broad activity in various xeno graft cancer models [86]. Dolly et al. recently reported in phase I study that this drug showed noticeable antitumor activity in MM patients at a generally well-tolerated dose [87].

GENE THERAPY

Another treatment option is under exploring by the genetic researchers to safely treat mesothelioma patients. Suicide gene therapy is one of the most promising forms of gene therapy for the treatment of MM. Clinical trials conducted at the University of Pennsylvania Medical Center shows that the suicide gene therapy is effective in reducing the size and severity among four of the 34 patients studied. Another type of gene therapy is under trial in which modified viruses are used to deliver immune system molecules called cytokines which direct and control immune response. These cytokines can help the immune system to mount an attack against cancer cells when introduced through gene therapy [63, 64].

Photodynamic Therapy

This is an option under trial, in which medical researchers seek to improve its efficacy and utilization in the treatment of mesothelioma. Researchers hope to develop photosensitizers that specifically target cancer cells and have more toxic reactions. They also hope to find a more effective ways of administering the necessary light, which can penetrate tissue and treat larger tumors [66].

Immunotherapy

The immune system plays a fundamental role in tumor development, growth and control. Mesothelioma appears to enjoy an "immune tolerance" state, although it is highly infiltrated by a population of immune cells [88]. Any decrease in cytotoxic T cells, antigen-presenting cells, natural killer lymphocytes, or increase in regulatory T cells, and production of immunoregulatory cytokines may contribute to the suppression of immune response [89, 90]. Reconstitution of the immune system to target tumor cells has become an attractive approach and one of the most active areas in mesothelioma research consequently [91].

Mesothelin is a cell-surface glycoprotein widely expressed in normal and malignant mesothelial cells and in other solid tumors [92]. It may be an important target for mesothelin-expressing tumors and a useful biomarker, [93] and may promote matrix metalloproteinase 9 expression in MM and tumor invasion [94].

Amatuximab (MORAb-009; Morphotek, Exton, PA, http://www.morphotek.com), a high-affinity monoclonal antibody toward mesothelin, has been evaluated in a phase I trial [95]. In 24 previously treated patients (including 13 with MM), amatuximab was well tolerated, and 11 patients had stable disease after receiving at least one cycle.

In a single-arm phase II study of amatuximab plus pemetrexed and cisplatin, Hassan et al. reported a partial RR of 39% ($n = 30$), and 51% ($n = 39$) had stable disease [96]. The same group has also investigated SS1P, a recombinant immunotoxin consisting of an antimesothelin antibody linked to a *Pseudomonas* exotoxin [97]. In a phase I trial, SS1P showed activity in heavily pretreated patients with mesothelin-expressing cancers and was well tolerated [98]. A major antitumor response was observed in 3 of 10 patients with advanced chemorefractory mesothelioma when SS1P was given together with immunosuppression in a recently published phase II study [99].

CRS-207 (Aduro BioTech, Berkeley, CA, http://www.adurobiotech.com) is a live-attenuated *Listeria* monocytogene vaccine designed to express mesothelin that was shown to be safe and to produce mesothelin-specific T- cell responses in a phase I trial that included five patients with MM [100].

Krug et al. designed a WT1 vaccine (WT1 protein is an oncogenic transcription factor commonly overexpressed in MM. Processed WT1 peptides can be presented to the immune system, making it an attractive target for T- cell-based immunotherapy [101]) and found it to be safe and effective in a pilot study [102].

This group is currently testing the vaccine in a randomized phase II trial in MM patients with minimal disease burden after multimodality therapy [103].

Dao et al. engineered a fully human "T cell receptor–like" monoclonal antibody, ESK1 [104], and found that ESK1 bound to several cancer cell lines (including mesothelioma) and primary leukemia cells with high avidity and they reported that it nearly cleared all leukemia in two mouse models without toxicity. These exciting preclinical data have positioned ESK1 to be tested further in clinical trials.

In normal epithelial cells, transforming growth factor β (TGF-β) is a promoter of cellular differentiation and a potent growth inhibitor [105]. However, tumor cells are often insensitive to this cytokine and can "utilize" TGF-β to promote host immunosuppression and tumor angiogenesis [106]. Significant levels of TGF-β are produced in MM cells lines and in primary MM tissues and pleural effusions [107, 108].

The first phase II trial of GC1008 (fresolimumab; Genzyme, Cambridge, MA, http://www.genzyme.com, which is a human monoclonal antibody capable of neutralizing all mammalian isoforms of TGF-β with high affinity [109]) in pretreated progressive MM was terminated, unfortunately, after only 13 enrollments when the manufacturer discontinued development of the antibody for oncological indications [110]. Although partial or complete radiographic responses were not observed, 3 patients showed stable disease at 3 months. Serum from 5 patients showed new or enhanced levels of antitumor antibodies, and these patients had increased median OS compared with those who did not show new or enhanced antitumor antibody levels (15 versus 7.5 months; $p < .03$).

Sterman et al. evaluated locally administered immunotherapy using two intrapleural doses of an adenoviral vector encoding human interferon-α (Ad.IFN-α2b), where five of nine patients showed evidence of tumor regression or disease stability in the pilot study [111]. Moreover, this group conducted a phase I/II trial involving repeated intrapleural "vaccination" with Ad.IFN-α2b concomitant with high-dose cyclooxygenase-2 inhibitor celecoxib, followed by standard first-line (pemetrexed-based) or second-line (gemcitabine-based) chemotherapy [112]. The disease control rate was 78% and the overall RR was 31%. Patients who received first-line chemotherapy ($n = 14$) had a median survival of 10.5 months, whereas patients with second- line chemotherapy ($n = 21$) had a median survival of 15.0 months. These promising results should be confirmed by randomized multicenter trials.

The antitumor activity of T cells can be inhibited by negative regulatory "checkpoint" proteins on the cell surface, such as programmed cell death 1 (PD1) and cytotoxic T-lymphocyte-associated protein 4 (CTLA4) [113]. Preclinical studies have demonstrated that CTLA4 blockage could augment endogenous responses to tumor cells, leading to tumor cell death [114].

Calabrò et al. evaluated tremelimumab (MedImmune, Gaithersburg, MD, https://www.medimmune.com), a human IgG2 monoclonal antibody to CTLA4, in patients with chemotherapy-resistant MM, in a recently published single-arm phase II study [115]. Although the study did not reach its primary endpoint which is a RR of 17%, the disease control rate was 31%. The median PFS was 6.2 with an OS of 10.7 months. Currently, a larger multicenter randomized phase II trial comparing tremelimumab to placebo in the second- or third-line setting is recruiting.

Another new approach called cancer vaccine is also aimed at getting the immune system to attack the cancer. In one approach, immune cells are removed from a patient's blood and treated in the lab to get them to react to tumor cells. The immune cells are then given back to the patient as blood transfusions, therefor, will initiate the body's immune system to attack the cancer.

Virus Therapies

Researchers are also studying the use of specially designed viruses to treat mesothelioma. This approach is still in the early phases of clinical trials.

These viruses can be put into the pleural space; hopefully, they can either infect and kill the cancer cells directly, or cause the immune system to attack the cancerous cells.

Several clinical trials are in progress, evaluating new ways to treat mesothelioma. It should be noted that peritoneal mesothelioma are classified as being clinically aggressive types of cancer. This means they can spread rapidly. In addition, the testicular type tends to recur within a few years, even in cases where tumors are surgically removed.

Prognosis

Malignant pleural mesothelioma has a poor prognosis in most patients, with a high mortality rate within 4 to 6 months. Some patients may survive 15 to 18 months with appropriate management and thorough follow-up. Postoperative tumor recurrence represents a critical prognostic factor, where the 5-year survivals have been rarely reported. Nevertheless, patients undergoing surgery may have slightly longer survival, despite the postoperative adverse events, including wound infection, postoperative bleeding, deep vein thrombosis, arrhythmias, air leak, respiratory failure, and myocardial infarction. Poor prognostic factors include age over 75-year, dyspnea and chest pain on presentation, elevated lactate dehydrogenase and low anemia on presentation, non-epithelial histology, poor performance status, and weight loss. [116].

REFERENCES

[1] Bridda A, Padoan I, Mencarelli R, and etal. Peritoneal Mesothelioma: A Review. *Med Gen Med.* 2007;9(2):32. [PubMed].

[2] Cunha P, Luz Z, Seves I. Malignant peritoneal mesothelioma – diagnostic and therapeutic difficulties. *Acta Med Port.* 2002;15: 383–386. [PubMed].

[3] Bianchi C, Bianchi T. Malignant mesothelioma: global incidence and relationship with asbestos. *Industrial Health.* 2007;45(3):379–387. [PubMed].

[4] Robinson BW, Lake RA. Advances in malignant mesothelioma. *N Engl J Med.* 2005;353:1591–1603. [PubMed].

[5] Teta MJ, Mink PJ, Lane E. US mesothelioma pattern 1973-2002: indicators of change and insight into background rate. *Eu J Cancer Prev.* 2008;17:525.

[6] Brigand C, Monneuse O, Mohamed F. Peritoneal mesothelioma treated by cytoreductive surgery and intraperitoneal hyperthermic chemotherapy: results of a prospective study. *Ann Surg Oncol.* 2006;13:405–412. [PubMed].

[7] Levy AD, Arnáiz J, Shaw JC, etal. From the archives of the AFIP: primary peritoneal tumors: imaging features with pathologic correlation. *Radiographics.* 2008;28(2):583.

[8] Abratt RP, White NW, Vorobiof DA. Epidemiology of mesothelioma--a South African perspective. *Lung Cancer.* 2005;49(Suppl 1):S13–15.

[9] Berry G, Roger J, Pooley FD. Mesotheliomas. Asbestos exposure and lung burden. In: Bignon J, Peto J, Saracci R, editors. Non occupational exposure to mineral fibers. *Lyon,* France: 1989. pp. 486–496. IARC scientific publication No 90.

[10] Selikoff IJ, Hammond EC, Seidman H. Latency of asbestos disease among insulation workers in the United States and Canada. *Cancer.* 1980;46:2736–2740. [PubMed].

[11] Mlika M, Lamzirbi O, Limam M, et al. Clinical and pathological profile of the pleural malignant mesothelioma: A retrospective study about 30 cases. *Rev Pneumol Clin.* 2018 Dec;74(6):427-435.

[12] Lanphear BP, Buncher CR. Latent period for malignant mesothelioma of occupational origin. *J Occup Med.* 1992;34:718–721. [PubMed].

[13] Carbone M, Ly BH, Dodson RF, et al.: Malignant mesothelioma: facts, myths, and hypotheses *J Cell Physiol.* 2012 Jan;227(1):44-58.

[14] Lisa Fayed: Asbestos and Cancer Risk, *American Cancer Society* 2015.

[15] Tward JD, Wendl MM, Shrieve DC, et al. Therisk of secondary malignancies over 30 years after the treatment of non-Hodgkin lymphoma. *Cancer.* 2006;107:108–115.

[16] Gibb H, Fulcher K, Nagarajan S, et al. Analyses of radiation and mesothelioma in the US Transuranium and Uranium Registries. *Am J. Public Health. 2013*;103: 710–716. [PMC free article] [PubMed].

[17] Comar M, Zanotta N, Pesel G, et al. Asbestos and SV40 in malignant pleural mesothelioma from a hyperendemic area of north-eastern Italy. *Tumori.* 2012;98:210–214. [PubMed].

[18] Cristaudo A, Foddis R, Vivaldi A, et al. SV40 enhances the risk of malignant mesothelioma among people exposed to asbestos: A molecular epidemiologic case-control study. *Cancer Res.* 2005; 65:3049–3052. [PubMed].

[19] Lundstig A, Dejmek A, Eklund C, et al. No detection of SV40 DNA in mesothelioma tissues from a high incidence area in Sweden. *Anticancer Res.* 2007;27: 4159–4161. [PubMed].

[20] Manfredi JJ, Dong J, Liu WJ, et al. Evidence against a role for SV40 in human mesothelioma. *Cancer Res.* 2005;65: 2602–2609. [PubMed].

[21] Carbone M, Ferris LK, Baumann F, et al. BAP1 cancer syndrome: Malignant mesothelioma, uveal and cutaneous melanoma, and MBAITs. *J Transl Med.* 2012;10: 179. [PubMed].

[22] Carbone M, Yang H, Pass HI, et al. BAP1 and cancer. *Nat Rev Cancer.* 2013;13:153–159. [PubMed].

[23] Testa JR, Cheung M, Pei J, et al. Germline BAP1 mutations predispose to malignant mesothelioma. *Nat Genet.* 2011;43:1022–1025. [PubMed].

[24] Bott M, Brevet M, Taylor BS, et al. The nuclear deubiquitinase BAP1 is commonly inactivated by somatic mutations and 3p21.1 losses in malignant pleural mesothelioma. *Nat Genet.* 2011;43:668–672 [PubMed].

[25] Lynne Eldridg. *Tips for improving lung cancer survival*, 2016.

[26] Ascoli V, Scalzo CC, Bruno C, Facciolo F, Lopergolo M, Granone P, Nardi F. Familial pleural malignant mesothelioma: clustering in three sisters and one cousin. *Cancer Lett.* 1998;130(1-2):203–207. [PubMed].

[27] Altekruse S, Kosary C, Krapcho M, et al., *SEER Cancer Statistics Review, 1975-2007*. National Cancer Institute; Bethesda, MD: 2010. http://seer.cancer.gov/csr/1975_2007/based on November 2009 SEER data submission, posted to the SEER web site.

[28] Aoe K, Hiraki A, Murakami T, et al., Infrequent existence of simian virus 40 large T antigen DNA in malignant mesothelioma in Japan. *Cancer Sci.* 2006;97(4):292–295.

[29] Ettinger DS, Wood DE, Akerley W, et al. NCCN Guidelines Insights: Malignant Pleural Mesothelioma. *J Natl Compr Canc Netw.* 2016 Jul;14(7):825-836. [PubMed].

[30] Plas E, Riedl CR, Pflüger H.: Malignant mesothelioma of the tunica vaginalis testis: review of the literature and assessment of prognostic parameters. *Cancer.* 1998;83:2437–2446.

[31] Fukunaga M. Well-differentiated papillary mesothelioma of the tunica vaginalis: a case report with aspirate cytological, immunohistochemically, and ultrastructural studies. *Pathol Res Pract.* 2010;206: 105–109.

[32] Trpkov K, Barr R, Kulaga A. et al. Mesothelioma of tunica vaginalis of "uncertain malignant potential": an evolving concept: case report and review of the literature. *Diagn Pathol.* 2011;6:78. [PubMed].

[33] Alesawi A.M., Levesque J., and Fradet V. Malignant esothelioma of the *tunica vaginalis* testis: with comprehensive review of literature and case report *Journal of Clinical Urology* 2013.

[34] Dodson RF, Graef R, Shepherd S, et al., Asbestos burden in cases of mesothelioma from individuals from various regions of the United States. *Ultrastructure. Pathol.* 2005;29:415–433. [Pub Med].

[35] Dodson RF, O'Sullivan M, Corn C, et al., Analysis of asbestos fiber burden in lung tissue from mesothelioma patients. *Ultrastruct. Pathol.* 1997;21:321–336. [PubMed].

[36] Rice DC, Stevens CW, Correa AM, et al. Outcomes after extrapleural pneumonectomy and intensity-modulated radiation therapy for malignant pleural mesothelioma. *Ann Thoracic. Surg.* 2007;84: 1685– 1692; discussion 1692–1693. [PubMed].

[37] Cho BC, Feld R, Leighl N, et al. A feasibility study evaluating Surgery for Mesothelioma After Radiation Therapy: The "SMART" approach for resectable malignant pleural mesothelioma. *J Thorac Oncol.* 2014;9:397–402. [PubMed].

[38] Dodson RF, O'Sullivan M, Brooks DR, Hammar SP. Quantitative analysis of asbestos burden in women with mesothelioma. *Am J Ind. Med.* 2003;43(2):188–195. [PubMed].

[39] Rodríguez D, Cheung MC, Housri N, et al., Malignant abdominal mesothelioma: defining the role of surgery. *J Surg. Oncol.* 2009; 99(1) [PubMed].

[40] Kusamura S, Younan R, Baratti D. Cytoreductive surgery followed by intraperitoneal hyperthermic perfusion: analysis of morbidity and mortality in 209 peritoneal surface malignancies treated with closed abdomen technique. *Cancer.* 2006;106:1144–1153. [PubMed].

[41] Gulmez I, Kart L, Buyukoglan H, et al. Evaluation of malignant mesothelioma in central Anatolia: A study of 67 cases. *Can Respir J.* 2004;11:287–290. [PubMed].

[42] Kadota K, Suzuki K, Sima CS, et al. Pleomorphic epithelioid diffuse malignant pleural mesothelioma: A clinicopathological review and conceptual proposal to reclassify as biphasic or sarcomatoid mesothelioma. *J. Thorac. Oncol.* 2011;6:896–904.

[43] Miettinen M, Limon J, Niezabitowski A, et al. Calretinin and other mesothelioma markers in synovial sarcoma: Analysis of antigenic similarities and differences with malignant mesothelioma. *Am J Surg. Pathol.* 2001;25:610–617.

[44] Creaney J, Christansen H, Lake R, et al. Soluble mesothelin related protein in mesothelioma. *J Thorac. Oncol.* 2006;1: 172–174. [PubMed].

[45] Schneider J, Hoffmann H, Dienemann H, et al. Diagnostic and prognostic value of soluble mesothelin-related proteins in patients

with malignant pleural mesothelioma in comparison with benign asbestosis and lung cancer. *J Thorac Oncol.* 2008;3:1317–1324.

[46] Pass HI, Levin SM, Harbut MR, et al. Fibulin-3 as a blood and effusion biomarker for pleural mesothelioma. *N Engl J Med.* 2012;367: 1417– 1427. [PubMed].

[47] Rai AJ, Flores RM, Mathew A, et al. Soluble mesohaline related peptides (SMRP) and osteopontin as protein biomarkers for malignant mesothelioma: Analytical validation of ELISA based assays and characterization at mRNA and protein levels. *Clin. Chem Lab Med.* 2010;48:271–278. [PubMed].

[48] Plathow C, Staab A, Schmaehl A, et al. Computed tomography, positron emission tomography, positron emission tomography/ computed tomography, and magnetic resonance imaging for staging of limited pleural mesothelioma: Initial results. *Invest Radiol.* 2008;43:737–744. [PubMed].

[49] Flores RM. Therole of PET in the surgical management of malignant pleural mesothelioma. *Lung Cancer.* 2005;49(suppl 1):S27–S32. [PubMed].

[50] Sørensen JB, Ravn J, Loft A, et al. Preoperative staging of mesothelioma by 18F-fluoro-2-deoxy-D-glucose positron emission tomography/computed tomography fused imaging and mediastinoscopy compared to pathological findings after extrapleural pneumonectomy. *Eur J Cardiothorac Surg.* 2008;34: 090–1096. [PubMed].

[51] Wilcox BE, Subramaniam RM, Peller PJ, et al. Utility of integrated computed tomography-positron emission tomography for selection of operable malignant pleural mesothelioma. *Clin Lung Cancer.* 2009;10:244–248. [PubMed].

[52] Rusch VW, Giroux D. Do we need a revised staging system for malignant pleural mesothelioma? Analysis of the IASLC database. *Ann Cardiothoracic Surg.* 2012;1:438–448. [PubMed].

[53] Rusch VW, Giroux D, Kennedy C, et al. Initial analysis of the International Association for the Study of Lung Cancer

mesothelioma database. *J. Thoracic Oncol.* 2012;7:1631–1639. [PubMed].

[54] Sugarbaker PH, Acherman YI, Gonzalez-Moreno S. Diagnosis and treatment of peritoneal mesothelioma: The Washington Cancer Institute experience. *Semin Oncol.* 2002;29:51–61.

[55] Sterman DH. Advances in management of mesothelioma. *Respirology.* 2005;10:266–283.

[56] Hesdorffer ME, Chabot JA, Keohan ML, et al. Combined resection, intraperitoneal chemotherapy, and whole abdominal radiation for the treatment of malignant peritoneal mesothelioma. *Am. J. Clin. Oncol.* 2008;31(1):49–54. [PubMed].

[57] Robinson BW, Musk AW, Lake RA. Malignant mesothelioma. *Lancet.* 2005;366: 397–408. [PubMed].

[58] Treasure T, Lang-Lazdunski L, Waller D, et al. Extra-pleural pneumonectomy versus no extra-pleural pneumonectomy for patients with malignant pleural mesothelioma: Clinical outcomes of the Mesothelioma and Radical Surgery (MARS) randomised feasibility study. *Lancet Oncol.* 2011;12:763–772. [PubMed].

[59] Zahid I, Sharif S, Routledge T, et al. Is pleurectomy and decortication superior to palliative care in the treatment of malignant pleural mesothelioma? *Interact Cardiovasc. Thorac Surg.* 2011;12:812–817. [PubMed].

[60] Teh E, Fiorentino F, Tan C, et al. A systematic review of lung-sparing extirpative surgery for pleural mesothelioma. *J R Soc Med.* 2011;104:69–80. [PMC free article] [PubMed].

[61] Rice D, Rusch V, Pass H, et al. Recommendations for uniform definitions of surgical techniques for malignant pleural mesothelioma: A consensus report of the International Association for the Study of Lung Cancer International Staging Committee and the International Mesothelioma Interest Group. *J Thorac Oncol.* 2011;6:1304–1312. [PubMed].

[62] Krug LM, Pass HI, Rusch VW, et al. Multicenter phase II trial of neoadjuvant pemetrexed plus cisplatin followed by extrapleural

pneumonectomy and radiation for malignant pleural mesothelioma. *J Clin Oncol.* 2009;27: 3007–3013. [PubMed].

[63] Ellis L, Atadja PW, Johnstone RW. Epigenetics in cancer: Targeting chromatin modifications. *Mol Cancer Ther.* 2009;8: 1409–1420. [PubMed].

[64] Paik PK, Krug LM. Histone deacetylase inhibitors in malignant pleural mesothelioma: Preclinical rationale and clinical trials. *J Thorac Oncol.* 2010;5:275–279. [PMC free article].

[65] Krug LM, Curley T, Schwartz L, et al. Potential role of histone deacetylase inhibitors in mesothelioma: Clinical experience with suberoylanilide hydroxamic acid. *Clin Lung Cancer.* 2006;7:257–261. [PubMed].

[66] Krug LM, Kindler H, Calvert H, et al. VANTAGE 014: Vorinostat (V) in patients with advanced malignant pleural mesothelioma (MPM) who have failed prior pemetrexed and either cisplatin or carboplatin therapy: A phase III, randomized, double-blind, placebo-controlled trial. *Eur J Cancer.* 2011;47:2–3.

[67] Remon J, Lianes P, Martínez S, et al. Malignant mesothelioma: New insights into a rare disease. *Cancer Treat Rev.* 2013;39:584–591. [PubMed].

[68] Kindler HL, Karrison TG, Gandara DR, et al. Multicenter, double-blind, placebo-controlled, randomized phase II trial of gemcitabine/cisplatin plus bevacizumab or placebo in patients with malignant mesothelioma. *Clin. Oncol.* 2012;30:2509–2515. [PMC free article] [PubMed].

[69] Dowell JE, Dunphy FR, Taub RN, et al. A multicenter phase II study of cisplatin, pemetrexed, and bevacizumab in patients with advanced malignant mesothelioma. *Lung Cancer.* 2012;77: 567–571. [PubMed].

[70] Zalcman G, Margery J, Scherpereel A, et al. IFCT-GFPC-0701 MAPS trial, a multicenter randomized phase II/III trial of pemetrexed-cisplatin with or without bevacizumab in patients with malignant pleural mesothelioma. *J Clin. Oncol.* 2010;28(suppl):7020a.

[71] Zalcman G, Mazieres J, Scherp ereel A, et al. IFCT-GFPC-0701 MAPS trial, a multicenter randomized phase III trial of pemetrexed-cisplatin with or without bevacizumab in patients with malignant pleural mesothelioma (MPM) *J. Clin. Oncol.* 2012;30 (suppl):TPS7112a.

[72] Hilberg F, Roth GJ, Krssak M, et al. BIBF 1120: Triple angiokinase inhibitor with sustained receptor blockade and good antitumor efficacy. *Cancer Res.* 2008;68:4774–4782. [PubMed].

[73] Mross K, Stefanic M, Gmehling D, et al. Phase I study of the angiogenesis inhibitor BIBF 1120 in patients with advanced solid tumors. *Clin Cancer Res.* 2010;16: 311–319. [PubMed].

[74] Reck M, Kaiser R, Mellemgaard A, et al. Docetaxel plus nintedanib versus docetaxel plus placebo in patients with previously treated non- small-cell lung cancer (LUME-Lung 1): A phase 3, double-blind, randomised controlled trial. *Lancet Oncol.* 2014;15:143–155. [PubMed].

[75] McClatchey AI, Fehon RG.: Merlin and the ERM proteins—regulators of receptor distribution and signaling at the cell cortex. *Trends Cell Biol.* 2009;19:198–206. [PubMed].

[76] Bianchi AB, Mitsunaga SI, Cheng JQ, et al. High frequency of inactivating mutations in the neurofibromatosis type 2 gene (NF2) in primary malignant mesotheliomas. *Proc Natl Acad Sci USA.* 1995;92:10854–10858. [PubMed].

[77] Sekido Y, Pass HI, Bader S, et al. Neurofibromatosis type 2 (NF2) gene is somatically mutated in mesothelioma but not in lung cancer. *Cancer Res.* 1995;55:1227–1231. [PubMed].

[78] Poulikakos PI, Xiao GH, Gallagher R, et al. Re-expression of the tumor suppressor NF2/merlin inhibits invasiveness in mesothelioma cells and negatively regulates FAK. *Oncogene.* 2006;25:5960–5968. [PubMed].

[79] Soria J-C, Gan HK, Arkenau H-T, et al. Phase I clinical and pharmacologic study of the focal adhesion kinase (FAK) inhibitor GSK2256098 in pts with advanced solid tumors. *J Clin Oncol.* 2012;30 (suppl):3000a.

[80] Katso R, Okkenhaug K, Ahmadi K, et al. Cellular function of phosphoinositide 3-kinases: Implications for development, homeostasis, and cancer. *Annu Rev Cell Dev Biol.* 2001;17:615–675. [PubMed].

[81] James MF, Han S, Polizzano C, et al. NF2/merlin is a novel negative regulator of mTOR complex 1, and activation of mTORC1 is associated with meningioma and schwannoma growth. *Mol Cell Biol.* 2009;29:4250–4261. [PubMed].

[82] López-Lago MA, Okada T, Murillo MM, et al. Loss of the tumor suppressor gene NF2, encoding merlin, constitutively activates integrin- dependent mTORC1 signaling. *Mol Cell Biol.* 2009;29:4235–4249. [PubMed].

[83] Garland LL, Ou S-H, Moon J, et al. SWOG 0722: A phase II study of mTOR inhibitor everolimus (RAD001) in malignant pleural mesothelioma (MPM) *J. Clin Oncol.* 2012;30(suppl):7083a.

[84] Wallin JJ, Edgar KA, Guan J, et al. GDC-0980 is a novel class I PI3K/mTOR kinase inhibitor with robust activity in cancer models driven by the PI3K pathway. *Mol Cancer Ther.* 2011;10: 2426–2436. [PubMed].

[85] Dolly S, Krug LM, Wagner AJ et al. Evaluation of tolerability and anti- tumor activity of GDC-0980, an oral PI3K/mTOR inhibitor, administered to patients with advanced malignant pleural mesothelioma (MPM). *Presented at: International Association for the Study of Lung Cancer 15th World Conference on Lung Cancer*; October 27–31, 2013; Sydney, Australia.

[86] Grégoire M. What's the place of immunotherapy in malignant mesothelioma treatments? *Cell Adhesion Migration.* 2010;4:153–161. [PubMed].

[87] Meloni F, Morosini M, Solari N, et al. Foxp3 expressing CD4+ CD25+ and CD8+CD28- T regulatory cells in the peripheral blood of patients with lung cancer and pleural mesothelioma. *Hum Immunol.* 2006;67:1–12. [PubMed].

[88] Solinas G, Germano G, Mantovani A, et al. Tumor-associated macrophages (TAM) as major players of the cancer-related inflammation. *J Leukoc Biol.* 2009;86:1065–1073. [PubMed].

[89] Bograd AJ, Suzuki K, Vertes E, et al. Immune responses and immunotherapeutic interventions in malignant pleural mesothelioma. *Cancer Immunol Immunother.* 2011;60:1509–1527. PubMed].

[90] Chang K, Pastan I. Molecular cloning of mesothelin, a differentiation antigen present on mesothelium, mesotheliomas, and ovarian cancers. *Proc Natl Acad Sci USA.* 1996;93:136–140. [PubMed].

[91] Hassan R, Ho M. Mesothelin targeted cancer immunotherapy. *Eur J Cancer.* 2008;44:46–53. [PubMed].

[92] Servais EL, Colovos C, Rodriguez L, et al. Mesothelin overexpression promotes mesothelioma cell invasion and MMP-9 secretion in an orthotopic mouse model and in epithelioid pleural mesothelioma patients. *Clin Cancer Res.* 2012;18:2478–2489. [PubMed].

[93] Hassan R, Cohen SJ, Phillips M, et al. Phase I clinical trial of the chimeric anti-mesothelin monoclonal antibody MORAb-009 in patients with mesothelin-expressing cancers. *Clin. Cancer Res.* 2010;16:6132–6138. [PubMed].

[94] Hassan R, Jahan TM, Kindler HL, et al. Amatuximab, a chimeric monoclonal antibody to mesothelin, in combination with pemetrexed and cisplatin in patients with unresectable pleural mesothelioma: Results of a multicenter phase II clinical trial. *J. Clin Oncol.* 2012;30 (suppl):7030a.

[95] Li Q, Verschraegen CF, Mendoza J, et al. Cytotoxic activity of the recombinant anti-mesothelin immunotoxin, SS1(dsFv)PE38, towards tumor cell lines established from ascites of patients with peritoneal mesotheliomas. *Anticancer Res.* 2004;24:1327–1335. [PubMed].

[96] Hassan R, Bullock S, Premkumar A, et al. Phase I study of SS1P, a recombinant anti-mesothelin immunotoxin given as a bolus i.v. infusion to patients with mesothelin-expressing mesothelioma, ovarian, and pancreatic cancers. *Clin. Cancer Res.* 2007;13:5144–5149. [PubMed].

[97] Hassan R, Miller AC, Sharon E, et al. Major cancer regressions in mesothelioma after treatment with an anti-mesothelin immunotoxin and immune suppression. *Sci Transl Med.* 2013;5:208 ra147. [PubMed].

[98] Le DT, Brockstedt DG, Nir-Paz R, et al. A live-attenuated Listeria vaccine (ANZ-100) and a live-attenuated Listeria vaccine expressing mesothelin (CRS-207) for advanced cancers: Phase I studies of safety and immune induction. *Clin Cancer Res.* 2012;18:858–868. [PMC free article] [PubMed].

[99] Thomas A, Hassan R. Immunotherapies for non-small-cell lung cancer and mesothelioma. *Lancet Oncol.* 2012;13:e301–e310. [PubMed].

[100] Krug LM, Dao T, Brown AB, et al. WT1 peptide vaccinations induce CD4 and CD8 T cell immune responses in patients with mesothelioma and non-small cell lung cancer. *Cancer Immunol Immunother.* 2010;59:1467–1479. [PMC free article] [PubMed].

[101] Krug L, Tsao AS, Kass S, et al. Randomized, double-blinded, phase II trial of a WT1 peptide vaccine as adjuvant therapy in patients with malignant pleural mesothelioma (MPM) *J Clin Oncol.* 2011;29(suppl):TPS139a.

[102] Dao T, Yan S, Veomett N, et al. Targeting the intracellular WT1 oncogene product with a therapeutic human antibody. *Sci Transl Med.* 2013;5:176ra33. [PubMed].

[103] Akhurst RJ, Hata A. Targeting the TGFβ signalling pathway in disease. *Nat Rev Drug Discov.* 2012;11:790–811. [PubMed].

[104] Massagué J. TGF beta in Cancer. *Cell.* 2008;134:215–230. [PubMed].

[105] Kumar-Singh S, Weyler J, Martin MJ, et al. Angiogenic cytokines in mesothelioma: A study of VEGF, FGF-1 and -2, and TGF beta expression. *J Pathol.* 1999;189:72–78. [PubMed].

[106] DeLong P, Carroll RG, Henry AC, et al. Regulatory T cells and cytokines in malignant pleural effusions secondary to mesothelioma and carcinoma. *Cancer Biol Ther.* 2005;4:342–346. [PubMed].

[107] Lonning S, Mannick J, McPherson JM. Antibody targeting of TGF-β in cancer patients. *Curr Pharm Biotechnol.* 2011;12:2176–2189. [PubMed].

[108] Stevenson JP, Kindler HL, Papasavvas E, et al. Immunological effects of the TGFβ-blocking antibody GC1008 in malignant pleural mesothelioma patients. *OncoImmunology.* 2013;2:e26218. [PubMed].

[109] Sterman DH, Haas A, Moon E, et al. A trial of intrapleural adenoviral- mediated Interferon-α2b gene transfer for malignant pleural mesothelioma. *Am J Respir Crit Care Med.* 2011;184:1395–1399 [PubMed].

[110] Sterman D, Alley E, Recio A et al. A pilot and feasibility trial evaluating two different chemotherapy regimens in combination with intrapleural adenoviral-mediated interferon-alpha (SCH 721015, Ad.hIFN-alpha2b) gene transfer for malignant pleural mesothelioma [abstract]. *Presented at: International Association for the Study of Lung Cancer 15th World Conference on Lung Cancer*; October 27–31, 2013; Sydney, Australia.

[111] Schreiber RD, Old LJ, Smyth MJ. Cancer immunoediting: Integrating immunity's roles in cancer suppression and promotion. *Science.* 2011;331:1565–1570. [PubMed].

[112] Grosso JF, Jure-Kunkel MN. CTLA-4 blockade in tumor models: An overview of preclinical and translational research. *Cancer Immun.* 2013;13:5. [PubMed].

[113] Calabrò L, Morra A, Fonsatti E, et al. Tremelimumab for patients with chemotherapy-resistant advanced malignant mesothelioma: An open- label, single-arm, phase 2 trial. *Lancet Oncol.* 2013;14:1104–1111. [PubMed].

[114] Jassem J, Ramlau R, Santoro A, et al. Phase III trial of pemetrexed plus best supportive care compared with best supportive care in previously treated patients with advanced malignant pleural mesothelioma. *J. Clin. Oncol.* 2008;26:1698–1704. [PubMed].

[115] Zucali PA, Ceresoli GL, Garassino I, et al. Gemcitabine and vinorelbine in pemetrexed-pretreated patients with malignant pleural mesothelioma. *Cancer.* 2008;112:1555–1561. [PubMed].

[116] Jain SV, Wallen JM. *Malignant Mesothelioma.*

Chapter 3

INFLAMMATORY AND IMMUNOLOGICAL ASPECTS IN THE SURGICAL MANAGEMENT OF MALIGNANT PLEURAL MESOTHELIOMA

Riccardo Tajè[1,*], Federico Tacconi[1], Roberto Fiorito[1], Alessandro Tamburrini[2] and Vincenzo Ambrogi[1]

[1]Department of Thoracic Surgery,
Policlinico Tor Vergata University, Rome, Italy
[2]Division of Thoracic Surgery, Southampton University Hospital, Southampton, UK

ABSTRACT

Malignant Pleural Mesothelioma is an aggressive cancer. Extrapleural pneumonectomy and extended pleurectomy/decortication are the two intentionally-radical surgical strategies, burdened with different complication rates. Both procedures fail to obtain true microscopic radical resection, achieving similar results in terms of disease-free and

---

[*] Corresponding Author's E-mail: ambrogi@uniroma2.it

overall survivals. Therefore, decision over the best surgical approach remains equivocal.

With the increasing knowledge regarding the influence of inflammation and immunity in carcinogenesis processes, several inflammatory markers gained prognostic values and currently affect therapeutic decisions and treatment strategies. Growing evidence supports the prognostic role of inflammatory markers such as neutrophils-to-lymphocytes ratio, platelets-to-lymphocytes ratio, albumin and C reactive protein in malignant pleural mesothelioma. Comprehensive and established prognostic scores including inflammatory markers may help surgeons to stratify patients pre-operatively.

Nonetheless, the effects of surgery on cancer immunity are debatable. Post-operative systemic inflammation may indeed hinder the immune system leading to immuno-tolerance, but on the contrary, surgical debulking may expose immunogenic epitope re-activating host defences against cancerous cells. A better knowledge and a more thorough understanding of this immunological balance could empower surgery with new significances, as surgery could both extirpate gross masses and function as an immunotherapy or radiotherapy booster in a multimodal treatment.

In this report we revise the role of the main inflammatory and immunological markers as prognostic indicators in malignant pleural mesothelioma. We also discuss the surgical effects on immune response against cancer.

INTRODUCTION

Surgery is a cornerstone within the multimodal management of malignant pleural mesothelioma but agreement regarding the best surgical strategy is lacking [1]. Extrapleural pneumonectomy and extended pleurectomy/decortication are the two intentionally curative surgeries. The former is an invasive procedure burdened with a high morbidity and mortality [2], which decrease when the operation is performed by very experienced surgeons [3]. The latter instead is a lung-sparing technique, aimed at grossly removing the tumor masses while preserving functional reserve [1]. The Mesothelioma and Radical surgery (MARS) trial questioned the safety of extrapleural pneumonectomy within the trimodal treatment strategy [2]. Nevertheless, the outcomes of the study were somehow controversial, due to the limited sample size and the higher-than-expected surgical-related mortality rate [1]. Novel comparative studies with larger sample size would be necessary to help identifying the best surgical strategy in patients with malignant pleural mesothelioma. Current guidelines suggest to tailor the choice between the two operations in highly selected patients who may benefit from a complete gross surgical cytoreduction. The surgical aggressiveness of extrapleural pneumonectomy compared to extended pleurectomy-decortication is obviously and noticeably higher, still both procedures fail to obtain a complete radical resection [1]. Hence, a careful assessment and balance of the risks of recurrence and the risks of major complications should guide the surgical choice. Histopathology, pulmonary function and availability of adjuvant or intraoperative chemotherapy can also affect the surgeon's choice, albeit the final decision is generally taken intraoperatively [1]. In this regard, the availability of new pre-operative prognostic factors may be of great support in the management of malignant pleural mesothelioma and help surgeons in selecting the best operative strategy. As showed in different reports, inflammation and its effects on the immune system greatly affect prognosis in cancer patients [4], as systemic inflammation hinders the immune response and reduces treatments' effectiveness [5]. In the setting of mesothelioma, several systemic inflammatory markers have been validated as negative prognostic factors and as predictive markers of response to treatment [4].

When considering extrapleural pneumonectomy and extended pleurectomy-decortication, it must be acknowledged that neither disease-free survival nor overall survival differ significantly between the procedures. Surgery is however still fundamental to give these patients a chance for an effective treatment [1]. Due to poor life expectancy of patients with mesothelioma, outcome goals other than disease free and overall survival, should be then taken into account. Immunological impairment caused by extensive surgical procedures can affect quality of life and treatment compliance in these patients [6, 7] and immune-suppression is also related with tumor relapse [5]. Thus, a better understanding of the inflammatory and immune-suppressive burden of surgery should be achieved to preserve quality of life, allow further adjuvant treatments and prevent recurrences.

PROGNOSTIC ROLE OF INFLAMMATORY AND IMMUNOLOGICAL MARKERS

Inflammation, immunity and cancer are strictly interdependent entities. Inflammation has a main role in cancer initiation, progression and metastasis, as it chronically damages tissues and hinders the immune response against tumor cells. Cancer causes its very own inflammatory response through necrosis and precarious angiogenesis and this type of chronic inflammation boosts cancer progression enhancing growth and neo-angiogenetic factors release from the tumor microenvironment [5]. Not surprisingly, in several malignancies local and systemic inflammatory markers showed prognostic value [8, 9]. Immunity exerts both pro- and anti-tumor effects and this ambiguous role may be affected by microenvironment alterations induced by surgical and pharmacological treatment and by cancer itself.

In mesothelioma, chronic inflammation plays a recognized and established etiopathogenic role [10]. Therefore, it is plausible that inflammatory markers may have prognostic significance. Hereafter, we will discuss the prognostic role of inflammatory cells, of ratios among inflammatory cells widely used in the clinical setting and of inflammation-based scores in the setting of mesothelioma.

BLOOD

Full blood cell count is widely available in the initial assessment of every patient. It normally entails absolute red blood cell count (RBC), white cell count (WBC), platelets count, hemoglobin and hematocrit. Red cells characteristics such as mean corpuscular volume (MCV) and red cells distribution width (RDW) or WBC differential are also generally included in the lab tests. Particularly, WBC count, WBC differential and platelets count have been associated with worse outcome in various cancers, and also in malignant pleural mesothelioma [11, 12]. Both leukocytosis and thrombocytosis, namely an excess in WBC or in platelets, reflect a chronic pro-inflammatory state [13], and it could partially explain their prognostic value in cancers.

Platelets Count

Platelets derive from megakaryocytes degranulation, which may be elicited by tumor mediators such as CD40 or tumor released cytokines. The larger is the release of inflammatory markers, the higher is the number of platelets elicited in the tumor microenvironment and in the peripheral blood. Thrombocytosis may therefore correlate with inflammation severity. Nonetheless, megakaryocytes degranulation itself releases mediators that enhance both tumor growth and leucocytes differentiation, thus megakaryocytes directly participate to tumor progression and immunological microenvironment development [11]. The role of thrombocytosis as prognostic marker in malignant pleural mesothelioma has been extensively explored. Billè et al. found platelets to be the only independent predictor of prognosis among all serum laboratory markers [14]. Nonetheless, Herndon et al. found platelet count >400.000/µL to be related with worse outcome with a 1.57 Relative Risk in the Cancer and Leukemia Group B (CALGB) score for malignant pleural mesothelioma prognosis [15].

White Blood Cell Count

The first evidences about the relationship between WBC count and prognosis in mesothelioma were found in 1998 by the European Organization for Research and Treatment of Cancer (EORCT) and

CALBG studies [15, 16]. In these studies, a higher WBC value was correlated to worse outcome. Particularly, in the CALBG study the prognostic sub-group with the worst outcome included patients with WBC≥15.6 and lower performance status. The role of WBC count has been further enhanced by the analysis of WBC differential and the implementation of ratios among WBC subtype that may reflect the pro-inflammatory status and the immune response withdrawal.

White Blood Cell Differential

White blood cell differential recognizes and counts the five WBC sub-population cells: neutrophils, lymphocytes, monocytes, eosinophils and basophils. Most of the studies investigating inflammatory burden in malignant disorders, evaluate the increment in the neutrophils absolute count (neutropilia) and the lymphocyte decrement (lymphocytopenia) as a sign of the patient's inflammatory and immunological status. Generally, both neutrophilia and lymphocytopenia suggest a decrease of the immune response. Neutrophilia has been related to the loss of the cytolytic ability of Natural Killer cells and cytotoxic lymphocyte leading to an ineffective protection against cancerous cells [17, 18]. Neutrophils releases growth-factors and enzymes capable to further stimulate tumor development [4]. Nonetheless, lymphocytes infiltrating tumor mass have been associated with better prognosis, [19-21], hence a decrease in lymphocytes count may prevent this beneficial effect.

Peripheral monocytes and their tissue infiltrating counterparts, tumor associated macrophages, have gained greater consideration in cancer development and progression [22]. The role of tumor associated macrophages hasn't been completely understood but they appear to enhance angiogenesis, tumor progression and immune-tolerance [23]. Generally, an increase in circulating monocytes reflects a higher tumor load and a higher density of tumor associated macrophages [24]. Nonetheless, higher monocytes alone were found to have a negative prognostic role in malignant pleural mesothelioma, independently from the histology sub-type [24].

Hemoglobin

Low hemoglobin level up to frank anemia are frequently observed in cancer and their origin is often multifactorial [25], entailing tumor bleeding and several other unknown causes generally included in the clinical spectrum named chronic illness anemia [26]. This condition may derive from cytokines-induced inhibition of the endogenous erythropoietin production [25]. Anemia has been associated with worse quality of life and prognosis in several malignant disorders [27, 28]. The prognostic role of anemia in mesothelioma has been initially described by Herndon et al. in the EORCT trial, [16] where anemia was related to a worse prognosis at univariate analysis. Subsequently, Kao et al. [29], found anemia to be independently associated with poor outcome in patients with mesothelioma.

Red Cell Distribution Width (RDW)

Circulating red cells have different volumes and RDW is a parameter commonly used in the management of anemia showing the heterogeneity of erythrocyte volume or anisocytosis. Consequently, a high RDW means that there are red blood cells of extremely different dimensions circulating. This may indicate an alteration in erythropoiesis or a deficit in erythrocyte homeostasis. Nonetheless, RDW has been associated with several diseases such as cancer and chronic inflammations. [30]. Abakay et al. showed that RDW has prognostic value in mesothelioma with a 2.77-fold increase in mortality rate and a significant decrease in mean survival time (8 vs 13.9 months) in patients with RDW > 20% versus < 20%. According to the author, the increased inflammatory status affected both RDW and survival [31].

Ratios

Neutrophil-to-Lymphocyte Ratio

Neutrophil-to-lymphocyte ratio (NLR) is an easy to obtain and cheap parameter derived from routine blood count, which has recently gained prognostic value in several malignancies [3]. Nonetheless, its relation with cancer prognosis hasn't still been fully elucidated. Hereafter we will try to briefly enlighten these blind spots. Namely, NLR is the result of the ratio been the absolute neutrophil count to the absolute lymphocyte count in the peripheral blood. Therefore, we can assume that a high NLR result from an increase in the neutrophil absolute count, a decrease in the lymphocytic absolute count or both. The impact on systemic inflammation of these conditions has been discussed above in this review but we can briefly summarize it as an immunological withdrawal due to cancer induced inflammation.

The prognostic role of NLR in mesothelioma has been extensively assessed. Kao and colleagues were the first to establish and validate this relation in different contexts [32, 33]. Abakay et al. [31] found a 1.6-fold increased mortality in patients with malignant pleural mesothelioma who had a NLR>3. Of particular interest for this review, is the prognostic role of NLR in patients undergoing extrapleural pneumonectomy. In this population, NLR with an optimal cut-off of 3 demonstrated a relation with prognosis with hazard risk of 1.72 NLR >3 vs NLR <3 [33]. Nonetheless, the prognostic role of NLR does not correlate with chemotherapy [29].

In addition, the NLR seems to have dynamic trend during disease progression, when fever, weight loss, sweat and other systemic inflammatory symptoms increase, as the disease progress [34, 35]. According to Kao et al, this may be the main reason of different cut-off values found to impact on prognosis inter [29]. The same author identified as the optimal cut-off a NLR>3 value in a study enrolling patients that were candidates for surgical resection (hence likely with disease at early stage) and a NLR>5 in another study enrolling patients with inoperable disease [32, 33].

Platelet-to-Lymphocyte Ratio

Similarly to the NLR, platelet-to-lymphocyte ratio (PLR) is easy to obtain and has shown prognostic role in various tumors, such as colorectal and pancreatic cancer [36, 37]. From a biological perspective, PLR physiopathology is comparable to NLR. As we discussed earlier in this review, platelets have a leading role in the tumor related-inflammation leading to cancer progression. Megakaryocyte degranulation releases growth factors for the cancer itself and for the immune cell differentiation. Nonetheless, platelets seem to have a role in the neo-angiogenetic process that characterizes tumor progression. Therefore, thrombocytosis enhances the inflammatory burden of the oncological disease, but it may also reveal the process of new blood vessel development during cancerous progression and metastasis [38]. The role of PLR in malignant pleural mesothelioma has been assessed in different papers [39, 40]. Onur et al, found a PLR>158 to be a significant prognostic factor in a small population of 36 patients with malignant pleural mesothelioma [19]. In the study conducted by Pinato et al, a PLR>300 was a significant prognostic factor only at univariate analysis. In the same study, the relation among inflammatory markers and neo-angiogenesis was investigated but the absolute count of platelets or PLR were not included in the analysis. Therefore, a direct evidence of the relation between platelet count or PLR and malignant pleural mesothelioma is still lacking. To the best of our knowledge, no studies have investigated the relation among PLR and prognosis after extended pleurectomy/decortication or extrapleural pneumonectomy.

Lymphocyte-to-Monocyte Ratio (LMR)

Lymphocyte to monocyte ratio is a novel prognostic marker in cancer. The use of this score has been validated especially for lung and pancreatic cancer [41, 42]. As we discussed earlier in this review, a low monocytes concentration reveals a lower tumor macrophage infiltration and a better prognosis. As it can be easily derived from the LMR equation, a high LMR indicates either an increase in lymphocyte or a decrease in circulating monocytes (or both) and it appears to correlate with more favourable prognosis. Conversely, low levels of LMR are associated with poor overall survival. Yamagishi et al. [43], found that a LMR <2.74 had a Hazard Risk 2.34 of death in patients with pleural mesothelioma. The mean survival of patients with a LMR lower then 2.74 was 5 months, while the mean survival of patients with a LMR higher than 2.74 was 14 months. In the subgroup analysis, the predictive value of LMR was significant when stratified by surgical intervention and no surgical intervention. This finding may lay the foundation of further studies investigating the role of LMR in the perioperative setting.

In a study conducted by Tanrikulu et al, patients with mesothelioma presenting a LMR <2.6 had a 1.8-fold increased mortality rate and LMR was the marker with the highest relation to prognosis compared to NLR, PLR and other inflammatory markers [44].

Osteopontin (OPN)

Early T lymphocyte activation-1 (Eta-1) or Osteopontin (OPN) is expressed in the early phases of type-1 immunity enhancement and its role is to potentiate macrophages activation through IL-12 while inhibiting IL-10 activation, thus allowing type 1 immunity differentiation [45]. Nonetheless, OPN also takes part in tissue remodelling and wound healing [46]. The role of OPN in cancer development has been investigated in vitro and in vivo [47]. Inducing the expression of OPN in mice lead to the development of more aggressive phenotype [47]. In lung cancer, an increase in OPN was related to stage of disease, relapse and immediate post-surgical inflammation, while decreasing of OPN could be observed weeks after surgery [48, 49].

In the setting of mesothelioma, the role of OPN has been assessed but confirmative studies are still lacking. Cappia et al. [50], demonstrated that OPN expression was significantly lower in long-term survival compared to short-term survival, with other studies reporting similar results as well Hollevoet et al. [51], demonstrated that patients with OPN values above 862.78 ng/ml had a significantly better survival than patients with OPN below this value, with an estimated median progression free survival of

14.3 months (95% CI= 8.5 – 20.1 months) compared to 5.6 months (95% CI= 84.4 – 6.8 months). In the same study, OPN values were related to radiological response to chemotherapy. Nonetheless, as in lung cancer, OPN was significantly higher immediately after extrapleural pneumonectomy and then decreased months after surgery. This finding may also corroborate the role OPN in tissue remodelling after surgery.

Prognostic Groups

As we discussed, systemic inflammation has a prominent role in the management of mesothelioma and several inflammatory markers and scores may help to predict prognosis. However, the actual utilization of this great amount of data in the clinical practice may be confusing, and it needs to be standardized within prognostic groups that may effectively help clinicians in the treatment choice. Therefore, different risk classification systems have been developed including clinical, pathological and radiological parameters in prognosis-stratified groups. Prognostic factors in their complexity will be discussed elsewhere in this book. Herein, we will highlight the role of inflammatory markers in these prognostic groups.

Cancer and Leukemia Group B

The Cancer and Leukemia Group B (CALGB) utilized performance status, age, hemoglobin level, presence of chest pain or weight loss and WBC to evaluate six prognostic groups. Patients with WBC higher than $15.6/\mu l$ and patients with worse performance status had the worst prognosis with a median survival of 1.4 months. In this scenario, the importance of WBC in prognosis of mesothelioma was again highlighted [15].

European Organization for Research and Treatment of Cancer (EORTC)

The European Organization for Research and Treatment of Cancer (EORTC) prognostic groups [16] included five variables: WBC count, performance status, certainty of histological diagnosis, histological subtype, and gender. Each variable was weighted as follows: prognostic score +0.55 for WBC count > 8.3 X 109/L, +0.60 for performance status 1 or 2, +0.52 when histological diagnosis was probable or possible, +0.67 for sarcomatoid subtype and +0.60 if male gender. Patients were then stratified into two risk classes. The low-risk class included patients with a comprehensive score ≤1.27 while the high-risk class entailed the remaining patients. Patients in the high-risk group had a RR of 2.9 (95% CI, 2.0 to 4.1%; P <.001) compared to the low-risk patients. The median survival was almost twice in the low risk versus the high-risk group (10.8 months vs 5.5 months).

Modified Glasgow Prognostic Score (mGPS)

The modified Glasgow Prognostic Score (mGPS) is an inflammatory based prognostic score validated in oncology, which takes into account the serum level of albumin and C reactive protein (CRP) [52]. The former is commonly used in clinical practice to evaluate the patient's nutritional status while the latter is a non-specific systemic inflammatory marker [52]. A decrease in albumin level has been generally associated with malnourishment, albeit newer trends in literature debunk the role of albumin in the nutritional assessment. Acute or chronic inflammation seems indeed to greatly affect albumin levels, reducing its specificity in the initial nutritional status evaluation [53]. C reactive protein is instead a non-specific inflammatory marker that may represent tumor cells death, and CRP increment has been associated with worse prognosis in several cancers [54]. Therefore, inflammation reduces significantly albumin levels while increasing CRP levels, resulting in higher values of mGPS. The mGPS has been validated as an independent prognostic indicator of stage of disease and response to treatment a stage in several non-thoracic cancers [55]. In malignant pleural mesothelioma, a mGPS≥1 has been associated with worse prognosis (Hazard risk=2.6; CI=1.6-4.2; p<0.001) [Pinato et al]. Particularly, 1-year OS was 72% for mGPS 0, 35% for mGPS 1 and 17% in patients with an mGPS 2, whereas the 2-year survival rate was 29, 17 and 4% for mGPS 0, 1 and 2, respectively.

Prognostic Risk Classification (PRC)

The Prognostic Risk Classification (PRC) System [56] is a novel prognostic system based on the histology subtype (epithelioid vs non-epithelioid), NLR, serum lactate de-hydrogenase and total lesion glycolysis. The latter can be derived from positron emission tomography as the metabolic tumor volume x the mean standard uptake value. These prognostic factors were chosen among sixteen of the most common risk factors for malignant mesothelioma. Particularly for the aim of this chapter, NLR greater than 5 demonstrated to have a hazard risk 1.6 (1.1-2.5); p=0.01. All prognostic factors had the same importance in the PRC system, defining a low-risk group with zero risk factors, a moderate-risk group counting only one risk factor and a high-risk group for patients depicting two or more risk factors.

EFFECTS OF INFLAMMATION ON QUALITY OF LIFE

We have previously described the role of inflammation in mesothelioma and the strategies to assess the inflammatory burden in order to establish prognostic models in the patients' stratification. Notwithstanding, mesothelioma has generally a dismal prognosis, therefore it may be of great interest to evaluate the effect of inflammation on other domains in patients' life, rather than survival. Inflammation greatly affects quality of life inducing several symptoms [57, 58]. Patients with high inflammatory burden complain of fatigue, allodynia, depression, fever and other invalidating symptoms limiting their everyday lives [57]. In malignant pleural mesothelioma, inflammatory markers such as NLR or CRP have been demonstrated to be directly associated with fatigue, anorexia and a generalized decline in quality of life [6]. In the same study, quality of life itself was shown to have prognostic value. Therefore, knowing the consequences of a high inflammatory burden may help the clinician.

Surgery Related Inflammatory and Immune Impairment in Cancer

Immunology and surgery seem to be far and incompatible spheres. As we discussed in the previous paragraphs, immunologic and inflammatory considerations may however help the surgeon in the choice of the surgical approach for mesothelioma (extrapleural pneumonectomy or extended pleurectomy/decortication). In this paragraph, we will discuss the controversial effect of surgery on the immune system. To a certain extent, surgery may affect the immune system by inducing a state of immunosuppression, leading to potential neoplastic relapses and infectious complications. Conversely surgical debulking may unreveal immunogenic epitope hidden in the neoplastic core.

The perioperative period entails an inevitable tissue damage. Surgery-related cellular damage, organ manipulation, tissue cauterization and vascular ligation inducing hypoperfusion are some of the events that contribute to post surgery inflammatory activation. All these events may release molecules like mitochondrial DNA or abnormal proteins resulting from cellular necrosis that initiate the inflammatory cascade. These pro-inflammatory molecules are called Damage Associated Molecular Pattern or DAMP molecules. DAMP molecules act similarly to microbial compounds sharing some of their pattern recognition receptors leading to cytokines transcription and immune response activation. Unexpectedly, post-surgical immune response is addressed more towards an immunosuppressing pattern [59]. The pathogenesis underlining post-surgical immune withdrawal has not been comprehensively understood. Particularly, IL-6 seems to play a central role in the immune modulation following surgery [60]. The signaling of IL-6 is commonly associated with STAT-3 pattern, which decreases the expression of the major histocompatibility complex among dendritic cells and impedes the presentation of the antigen [61]. Nonetheless, IL-6 has been associated with a reduced IL-12 secretion, hindering the proliferation of CD4 and CD8 T cells and the interferon release [62]. Surgery also activates the hypothalamic-pituitary-adrenal axis leading to cortisol release that participates to the immune withdrawal [63]. Under this perspective, also the anesthesiologic management has a role in the immunologic burden, since anesthesia may activate adrenergic inflammatory pathway increasing cortisol release and obstructing the immune cells towards the tumor mass [63].

Nonetheless, surgical invasiveness seems to be related to the magnitude of cytokines response [64].

This immunosuppressive state can elucidate why patients undergoing extensive surgical resections are at high risk for infectious complications. [60, 65]. Therefore, it seems reasonable to question whether post-surgical immune-depression can boost cancer relapse [66].

In thoracic surgery, the effects of thoracotomy versus thoracoscopy upon inflammation have been evaluated in lung cancer. As expected, thoracoscopy has less impact on inflammatory response preserving the immune system [66]. Nonetheless, how the different approaches affect disease-free survival is not clear. A minimally invasive approach through thoracoscopy has been associated with less local recurrences [67] but it was found not to predict significantly longer disease-free survival [68].

In malignant pleural mesothelioma the immunological effects of surgery are completely unknown. As we discussed, disease-free survival and overall survival do not differ significantly between the two established surgical procedures [1]. One of the most significant exception is a retrospective analysis showing that pleurectomy/decortication predicted a longer disease-free survival versus extrapleural pneumonectomy but selection bias could not be excluded [69]. Therefore, as differences in disease free survival among the two procedures are unclear, it is difficult to weight the immunological effects of surgery in the time to recurrence patterns. Nonetheless, as we discussed, surgery is unable to obtain a true microscopic radical resection. Whether the remaining cells may take advantage of the surgical transitory immunosuppressive status, cytoreductive surgery can reveal tumor epitopes hidden from the immune system [63]. Surgery creates the chance to reset the tumor induced immune-tolerance toward cancerous cells enhancing chemotherapy and immunotherapy effects [70]. This may explain the success of the multimodal treatment strategies and the crucial role of surgery in this context. Future studies can integrate strategies to reduce post-surgical and anesthesiologic immunodepression.

CONCLUSION

Immunology can have a crucial role in surgery. The pro-inflammatory status following cancer exerts an inhibitory effect on the immune system interfering with prognosis. Different prognostic scores based on serum inflammatory and immune markers have been developed to help stratify patients in risk classes. Recognizing the relevance of the novel prognostic scores may assist the surgeon in choosing between extrapleural pneumonectomy and pleurectomy/decortication. Nonetheless, surgeon should be aware of the surgically-induced immunosuppressive status following invasive procedures and of the ability of surgery to reactivate immunity toward the cancerous cells.

REFERENCES

[1] National Comprehensive Cancer Network. *Malignant pleural mesothelioma* (Version 1.2021).

[2] Treasure T, Lang-Lazdunski L, Waller D, Bliss JM, Tan C, Entwisle J, Snee M, O'Brien M, Thomas G, Senan S, O'Byrne K, Kilburn LS, Spicer J, Landau D, Edwards J, Coombes G, Darlison L, Peto J. 2011. MARS trialists. Extra-pleural pneumonectomy versus no extra-pleural pneumonectomy for patients with malignant pleural mesothelioma: clinical outcomes of the Mesothelioma and Radical Surgery (MARS) randomised feasibility study. *Lancet Oncol* 12: 763-72. doi: 10.1016/S1470-2045(11)70149-8.

[3] Sugarbaker DJ, Wolf AS, Chirieac LR, Godleski JJ, Tilleman TR, Jaklitsch MT, Bueno R, Richards WG. 2011 Clinical and pathological features of three-year survivors of malignant pleural mesothelioma following extrapleural pneumonectomy. *Eur J Cardiothorac Surg* 40: 298-303. doi: 10.1016/j.ejcts.2010.12.024.

[4] Templeton AJ, McNamara MG, Šeruga B, Vera-Badillo FE, Aneja P, Ocaña A, Leibowitz-Amit R, Sonpavde G, Knox JJ, Tran B, Tannock IF, Amir E. 2014. Prognostic role of neutrophil-to-lymphocyte ratio in solid tumors: a systematic review and meta-analysis. *J Natl Cancer Inst* 29: 106-124. doi: 10.1093/jnci/dju124.

[5] Grivennikov SI, Greten FR, Karin M. 2010. Immunity, inflammation, and cancer. *Cell* 19; 140: 883-99. doi. 10.1016%2Fj.cell.2010.01.025.

[6] Kao SC, Vardy J, Harvie R, Chatfield M, van Zandwijk N, Clarke S, Pavlakis N. 2013. Health-related quality of life and inflammatory markers in malignant pleural mesothelioma. *Support Care Cancer* 21:697-705. doi: 10.1007/s00520-012-1569-6.

[7] Opitz I, Weder W. 2017. A nuanced view of extrapleural pneumonectomy for malignant pleural mesothelioma. *Ann Transl Med* 5: 237. doi: 10.21037/atm.2017.03.88.

[8] Al-Shibli KI, Donnem T, Al-Saad S, Persson M. Bremnes RM, Busund LT. 2008. Prognostic effect of epithelial and stromal lymphocyte infiltration in non-small cell lung cancer. *Clin Cancer Res* 14: 5220-7. doi: 10.1158/1078-0432.CCR-08-0133.

[9] McMillan DC, Crozier JE, Canna K, Angerson WJ, McArdle CS. 2007. Evaluation of an inflammation-based prognostic score (GPS) in patients undergoing resection for colon and rectal cancer. *Int J Colorectal Dis* 22:881-6. doi: 10.1007/s00384-006-0259-6.

[10] Gaudino G, Xue J, Yang H. 2020. How asbestos and other fibers cause mesothelioma. *Transl Lung Cancer Res* 9: S39-S46. doi: 10.21037/tlcr.2020.02.01.

[11] Cihan YB, Ozturk A, Mutlu H. 2014. Relationship between prognosis and neutrophil: lymphocyte and platelet:lymphocyte ratios

in patients with malignant pleural mesotheliomas. *Asian Pac J Cancer Prev* 15: 2061-7. doi: 10.7314/apjcp.2014.15.5.2061.

[12] Edwards JG, Abrams KR, Leverment JN, Spyt TJ, Waller DA, O'Byrne KJ. 2000. Prognostic factors for malignant mesothelioma in 142 patients: validation of CALGB and EORTC prognostic scoring systems. *Thorax* 55: 731-5. doi: 10.1136/thorax.55.9.731. PMID: 10950889.

[13] Klinger MH, Jelkmann W. 2002. Role of blood platelets in infection and inflammation. *J Interferon Cytokine Res* 22: 913-22. doi: 10.1089/10799900260286623.

[14] Billé A, Krug LM, Woo KM, Rusch VW, Zauderer MG. 2016. Contemporary Analysis of Prognostic Factors in Patients with Unresectable Malignant Pleural Mesothelioma. *J Thorac Oncol* 11: 249-55. doi: 10.1016/j.jtho.2015.10.003.

[15] Herndon JE II, Green MR, Chahinian AP, Corson JM, Suzuki Y, Vogelzang NJ. 1998. Factors predictive of survival among 337 patients with mesothelioma treated between 1984 and 1994 by the Cancer and Leukemia Group B. *Chest* 113: 723–731. doi: 10.1378/chest.113.3.723.

[16] Curran D, Sahmoud T, Therasse P, van Meerbeeck J, Postmus PE, Giaccone G. 1998. Prognostic factors in patients with pleural mesothelioma: the European Organization for Research and Treatment of Cancer experience. *J Clin Oncol* 16: 145–152. doi: 10.1200/JCO.1998.16.1.145.

[17] Petrie HT, Klassen LW, Kay HD. 1985. Inhibition of human cytotoxic T lymphocyte activity in vitro by autologous peripheral blood granulocytes. *J Immunol* 134: 230–234.

[18] el-Hag A, Clark RA. 1987. Immunosuppression by activated human neutrophils. Dependence on the myeloperoxidase system. *J Immunol* 139: 2406–2413.

[19] Loi S, Sirtaine N, Piette F, Salgado R, Viale G, Van Eenoo F, Rouas G, Francis P, Crown JP, Hitre E, de Azambuja E, Quinaux E, Di Leo A, Michiels S, Piccart MJ, Sotiriou C. 2013. Prognostic and predictive value of tumor-infiltrating lymphocytes in a phase III

randomized adjuvant breast cancer trial in node-positive breast cancer comparing the addition of docetaxel to doxorubicin with doxorubicin-based chemotherapy: BIG 02-98. *J Clin Oncol* 31: 860-7. doi: 10.1200/JCO.2011.41.0902.

[20] Gooden MJ, de Bock GH, Leffers N, Daemen T, Nijman HW. 2011. The prognostic influence of tumour-infiltrating lymphocytes in cancer: a systematic review with meta-analysis. *Br J Cancer* 105: 93–103. doi: 10.1038/bjc.2011.189.

[21] Denkert C, Loibl S, Noske A, Roller M, Müller BM, Komor M, Budczies J, Darb-Esfahani S, Kronenwett R, Hanusch C, von Törne C, Weichert W, Engels K, Solbach C, Schrader I, Dietel M, von Minckwitz G. 2010. Tumor-associated lymphocytes as an independent predictor of response to neoadjuvant chemotherapy in breast cancer. *J Clin Oncol* 28: 105-13. doi: 10.1200/JCO.2009.23.7370.

[22] Lievense LA, Bezemer K, Aerts JG, Hegmans JP. 2018. Tumor-associated macrophages in thoracic malignancies. *Lung Cancer* 80: 256–262. doi: 10.1016/j.lungcan.2013.02.017.

[23] Pollard JW. 2004. Tumour-educated macrophages promote tumour progression and metastasis, *Nat. Rev. Cancer* 4: 71–78. doi: 10.1038/nrc1256.

[24] Burt BM, Rodig SJ, Tilleman TR, Elbardissi AW, Bueno R, Sugarbaker DJ. 2011. Circulating and tumor-infiltrating myeloid cells predict survival in human pleural mesothelioma. *Cancer* 117: 5234–5244. doi: 10.1016/j.jtcvs.2014.03.011.

[25] Abdel-Razeq H, Hashem H. 2020. Recent update in the pathogenesis and treatment of chemotherapy and cancer induced anemia. *Crit Rev Oncol Hematol* 145: 102837. doi: 10.1016/j.critrevonc.2019.102837.

[26] Cullis J. 2013. Anaemia of chronic disease. *Clin Med (Lond)* 13: 193-6. doi: 10.7861/clinmedicine.13-2-193.

[27] Shrivastava S, Mahantshetty U, Engineer R, Chopra S, Hawaldar R, Hande V, Kerkar RA, Maheshwari A, Shylasree TS, Ghosh J, Bajpai J, Gurram L, Gulia S, Gupta S; Gynecologic Disease Management Group. 2018. Cisplatin Chemoradiotherapy vs Radiotherapy in FIGO

Stage IIIB Squamous Cell Carcinoma of the Uterine Cervix: A Randomized Clinical Trial. *JAMA Oncol* 4: 506-513.

[28] Curt GA. 2000. The impact of fatigue on patients with cancer: overview of FATIGUE 1 and 2. *Oncologist* 2: 9-12. doi: 10.1634/the oncologist.5-suppl_2-9.

[29] Kao SC, Vardy J, Chatfield M, Corte P, Pavlakis N, Clarke C, van Zandwijk N, Clarke S. 2013. Validation of prognostic factors in malignant pleural mesothelioma: a retrospective analysis of data from patients seeking compensation from the New South Wales Dust Diseases Board. *Clin Lung Cancer* 14: 70-7. doi: 10.1016/j.cllc. 2012.03.011.

[30] Salvagno GL, Sanchis-Gomar F, Picanza A, Lippi G. 2015. Red blood cell distribution width: A simple parameter with multiple clinical applications. *Crit Rev Clin Lab Sci* 52: 86-105. doi: 10.3109/10408363.2014.992064.

[31] Abakay O, Tanrikulu AC, Palanci Y, Abakay A. 2014. The value of inflammatory parameters in the prognosis of malignant mesothelioma. *J Int Med Res* 42: 554-65. doi: 10.1177/0300060 513504163.

[32] Kao SC, Pavlakis N, Harvie R, Vardy JL, Boyer MJ, van Zandwijk N, Clarke SJ. 2010. High blood neutrophil-to-lymphocyte ratio is an indicator of poor prognosis in malignant mesothelioma patients undergoing systemic therapy. *Clin Cancer Res* 16: 5805-13. doi: 10.1158/1078-0432.CCR-10-2245.

[33] Kao SC, Klebe S, Henderson DW, Reid G, Chatfield M, Armstrong NJ, Yan TD, Vardy J, Clarke S, van Zandwijk N, McCaughan B. 2011. Low calretinin expression and high neutrophil-to-lymphocyte ratio are poor prognostic factors in patients with malignant mesothelioma undergoing extrapleural pneumonectomy. *J Thorac Oncol* 6: 1923-9. doi: 10.1097/JTO.0b013e31822a3740.

[34] Nowak AK, Stockler MR, Byrne MJ. 2004. Assessing quality of life during chemotherapy for pleural mesothelioma: feasibility, validity, and results of using the European Organization for Research and Treatment of Cancer core quality of life questionnaire and lung

cancer module. *J Clin Oncol* 22:3172-80. doi: 10.1200/JCO.2004. 09.147.

[35] Robinson BW, Musk AW, Lake RA. 2005. Malignant mesothelioma. *Lancet* 366: 397-408. doi: 10.1016/S0140-6736(05)67025-0.

[36] Kwon HC, Kim SH, Oh SY, Lee S, Lee JH, Choi HJ, Park KJ, Roh MS, Kim SG, Kim HJ, Lee JH. 2012. Clinical significance of preoperative neutrophil-lymphocyte versus platelet-to-lymphocyte ratio in patients with operable colorectal cancer. *Biomarkers* 17: 216-22. doi: 10.3109/1354750X.2012.656705.

[37] Smith RA, Bosonnet L, Raraty M, Sutton R, Neoptolemos JP, Campbell F, Ghaneh P. 2009. Preoperative platelet-lymphocyte ratio is an independent significant prognostic marker in resected pancreatic ductal adenocarcinoma. *Am J Surg* 197(4): 466-72. doi: 10.1016/ j.amjsurg.2007.12.057.

[38] Sierko E, Wojtukiewicz MZ. 2004. Platelets and angiogenesis in malignancy. *Semin Thromb Hemost* 30: 95-108. doi: 10.1055/s-2004-822974.

[39] Tural Onur S, Sokucu SN, Dalar L, Iliaz S, Kara K, Buyukkale S, Altin S. 2016. Are neutrophil/lymphocyte ratio and platelet/lymphocyte ratio reliable parameters as prognostic indicators in malignant mesothelioma? *Ther Clin Risk Manag* 12: 651-6. doi: 10.2147%2FTCRM.S104077.

[40] Pinato DJ, Mauri FA, Ramakrishnan R, Wahab L, Lloyd T, Sharma R. 2012. Inflammation-based prognostic indices in malignant pleural mesothelioma. *J Thorac Oncol* 7: 587-94. doi: 10.1097/JTO.0b013 e31823f45c1.

[41] Lin GN, Peng JW, Xiao JJ, Liu DY, Xia ZJ. 2014. Prognostic impact of circulating monocytes and lymphocyte-to-monocyte ratio on previously untreated metastatic non-small cell lung cancer patients receiving platinum-based doublet. *Med Oncol* 31: 70. doi: 10.1007/s12032-014-0070-0.

[42] Fujiwara Y, Misawa T, Shiba H, Shirai Y, Iwase R, Haruki K, Furukawa K, Futagawa Y, Yanaga K. 2014. Postoperative peripheral absolute blood lymphocyte-to-monocyte ratio predicts therapeutic

outcome after pancreatic resection in patients with pancreatic adenocarcinoma. *Anticancer Res* 34: 5133-5138.

[43] Yamagishi T, Fujimoto N, Nishi H, Miyamoto Y, Hara N, Asano M, Fuchimoto Y, Wada S, Kitamura K, Ozaki S, Kishimoto T. 2015. Prognostic significance of the lymphocyte-to-monocyte ratio in patients with malignant pleural mesothelioma. *Lung Cancer* 90: 111-7. doi: 10.1016/j.lungcan.2015.07.014.

[44] Tanrikulu AC, Abakay A, Komek H, Abakay O. 2016. Prognostic value of the lymphocyte-to-monocyte ratio and other inflammatory markers in malignant pleural mesothelioma. *Environ Health Prev Med* 21: 304-311. doi: 10.1007/s12199-016-0530-6.

[45] Ashkar S, Weber GF, Panoutsakopoulou V, Sanchirico ME, Jansson M, Zawaideh S, Rittling SR, Denhardt DT, Glimcher MJ, Cantor H. 2000. Eta-1 (osteopontin): an early component of type-1 (cell-mediated) immunity. *Science* 287: 860-4. doi: 10.1126/science.287.5454.860.

[46] Liaw L, Birk DE, Ballas CB, Whitsitt JS, Davidson JM, Hogan BL. 1998, Altered wound healing in mice lacking a functional osteopontin gene (spp1). *J Clin Invest* 101: 1468-78. doi: 10.1172/JCI2131.

[47] Denhardt DT, Guo X. 1993. Osteopontin: A protein with diverse functions. *Faseb J* 7: 1475-1482.

[48] Chang YS, Kim HJ, Chang J, Ahn CM, Kim SK, Kim SK. 2007. Elevated circulating level of osteopontin is associated with advanced disease state of non-small cell lung cancer. *Lung Cancer* 57: 373-380. doi: 10.1016/j.lungcan.2007.04.005.

[49] Blasberg JD, Pass HI, Goparaju CM, Flores RM, Lee S, Donington JS. 2010. Reduction of elevated plasma osteopontin levels with resection of non-small-cell lung cancer. *J Clin Oncol* 28: 936-41. doi: 10.1200/JCO.2009.25.5711.

[50] Cappia S, Righi L, Mirabelli D, Ceppi P, Bacillo E, Ardissone F, Molinaro L, Scagliotti GV, Papotti M. 2008. Prognostic role of osteopontin expression in malignant pleural mesothelioma. *Am J Clin Pathol* 130: 58-64. doi: 10.1309/TWCQV536WWRNEU51.

[51] Hollevoet K, Nackaerts K, Gosselin R, De Wever W, Bosquée L, De Vuyst P, Germonpré P, Kellen E, Legrand C, Kishi Y, Delanghe JR, van Meerbeeck JP. 2011. Soluble mesothelin, megakaryocyte potentiating factor, and osteopontin as markers of patient response and outcome in mesothelioma. *J Thorac Oncol* 6: 1930-7. doi: 10.1097/JTO.0b013e3182272294.

[52] McMillan DC. 2008. An inflammation-based prognostic score and its role in the nutrition-based management of patients with cancer. *Proc Nutr Soc* 67: 257-62. doi: 10.1017/S0029665108007131.

[53] Eckart A, Struja T, Kutz A, Baumgartner A, Baumgartner T, Zurfluh S, Neeser O, Huber A, Stanga Z, Mueller B, Schuetz P. 2020. Relationship of Nutritional Status, Inflammation, and Serum Albumin Levels during Acute Illness: A Prospective Study. *Am J Med* 133: 713-722.e7. doi: 10.1016/j.amjmed.2019.10.031.

[54] Allin KH, Nordestgaard BG. 2011. Elevated C-reactive protein in the diagnosis, prognosis, and cause of cancer. *Crit Rev Clin Lab Sci* 48: 155-70. doi: 10.3109/10408363.2011.599831.

[55] Leitch EF, Chakrabarti M, Crozier JEM, McKee RF, Anderson JH, Horgan PG & McMillan DC. 2007. Comparison of the prognostic value of selected markers of the systemic inflammatory response in patients with colorectal cancer. *Br J Cancer* 97: 1266–1270. doi: 10.1038/sj.bjc.6604027.

[56] Doi H, Kuribayashi K, Kitajima K, Yamakado K, Kijima T. 2020. Development of a Novel Prognostic Risk Classification System for Malignant Pleural Mesothelioma. *Clin Lung Cancer* 21: 66-74.e2.

[57] Kelley K, Bluthe R, Dantzer R, Zhou JH, Shen WH, Johnson RW, Broussard SR. 2003. Cytokine-induced sickness behavior. *Brain Behav Immun* 17: S112–S118. doi: 10.1016/s0889-1591(02)00077-6.

[58] Seruga B, Zhang H, Bernstein LJ, Tannock IF. 2008. Cytokines and their relationship to the symptoms and outcome of cancer. *Nat Rev Cancer* 8: 887–899. doi: 10.1038/nrc2507.

[59] O'Dwyer MJ, Owen HC, Torrance HDT. 2015. The perioperative immune response. *Current Opinion in Critical Care* 21: 336–342. doi: 10.1097/MCC.0000000000000213.

[60] Mokart D, Capo C, Blache JL, Delpero JR, Houvenaeghel G, Martin C, Mege JL. 2002. Early postoperative compensatory anti-inflammatory response syndrome is associated with septic complications after major surgical trauma in patients with cancer. *Br J Surg* 89: 1450–1456. doi: 10.1046/j.1365-2168.2002.02218.x.

[61] Kitamura H, Kamon H, Sawa S, Park SJ, Katunuma N, Ishihara K, Murakami M, Hirano T. 2005. IL-6-STAT3 controls intracellular MHC class II alphabeta dimer level through cathepsin S activity in dendritic cells. *Immunity* 23: 491–502. doi: 10.1016/j.immuni.2005.09.010.

[62] Ohno Y, Kitamura H, Takahashi N, Ohtake J, Kaneumi S, Sumida K, Homma S, Kawamura H, Minagawa N, Shibasaki S, Taketomi A. 2016. IL-6 downregulates HLA class II expression and IL-12 production of human dendritic cells to impair activation of antigenspecific CD4(þ) T cells. *Cancer Immunol Immunother* 65: 193–204. doi: 10.1007/s00262-015-1791-4.

[63] Dubowitz JA, Sloan EK, Riedel BJ. 2018. Implicating anaesthesia and the perioperative period in cancer recurrence and metastasis. *Clin Exp Metastasis* 35: 347-358. doi: 10.1007/s10585-017-9862-x.

[64] Veenhof A, Sietses C, Von Blomberg B, Van Hoogstraten I, Vd Pas M, Meijerink W, Vd Peet D, Vd Tol M, Bonjer H, Cuesta M. 2011. The surgical stress response and postoperative immune function after laparoscopic or conventional total mesorectal excision in rectal cancer: a randomized trial. *Int J Colorectal Dis* 26: 53–59. doi: 10.1007/s00384-010-1056-9.

[65] Velasco E, Thuler LC, Martins CA, Dias LM, Conalves VM. 1996. Risk factors for infectious complications after abdominal surgery for malignant disease. *Am J Infect Control* 24:1-6. doi: 10.1016/s0196-6553(96)90046-2.

[66] Ng CS, Whelan RL, Lacy AM, Yim AP. 2005. Is minimal access surgery for cancer associated with immunologic benefits? *World J Surg* 29: 975–81. doi: 10.1177/0218492309338100.

[67] Higuchi M, Yaginuma H, Yonechi A, Kanno R, Ohishi A, Suzuki H, Gotoh M. 2014. Long-term outcomes after video-assisted thoracic

surgery (VATS) lobectomy versus lobectomy via open thoracotomy for clinical stage IA non-small cell lung cancer. *J Cardiothorac Surg* 17; 9:88. doi: 10.1186/1749-8090-9-88.

[68] Motono N, Iwai S, Iijima Y, Usuda K, Uramoto H. 2020. Operative invasiveness does not affect the prognosis of patients with non-small cell lung cancer. *BMC Pulm Med* 20: 265. doi: 10.1186/s12890-020-01264-x.

[69] Flores RM, Pass HI, Seshan VE, Dycoco J, Zakowski M, Carbone M, Bains MS, Rusch VW. 2008. Extrapleural pneumonectomy versus pleurectomy/decortication in the surgical management of malignant pleural mesothelioma: results in 663 patients. *J Thorac Cardiovasc Surg* 135: 620-6. doi: 10.1016/j.jtcvs.2007.10.054.

[70] Broomfield S, Currie A, van der Most RG, Brown M, van Bruggen I, Robinson BW, Lake RA. 2005. Partial, but not complete, tumor-debulking surgery promotes protective antitumor memory when combined with chemotherapy and adjuvant immunotherapy. *Cancer Res* 65: 7580-4. doi: 10.1158/0008-5472.CAN-05-0328.

BIOGRAPHICAL SKETCH

Vincenzo Ambrogi

Affiliation: Associate Professor of Thoracic Surgery at Tor Vergata University and Responsible of the Unit of Thoracic endoscopy and video-thoracoscopy at Policlinico Tor Vergata

Education: Prof. Ambrogi earned his medical degree Cum Laude from Perugia University. He trained in General Surgery and served as Resident at Policlinico Umberto I in Rome obtaining here the Italian Board in General Surgery. Thereafter he started a new postgraduate course in Thoracic Surgery serving as resident at St. Eugenio Hospital of Rome under his mentor Prof. Tommaso Claudio Mineo obtaining the Italian

Board of Thoracic Surgery at University of Rome La Sapienza with highest honors.

Research and Professional Experience: Thereafter he earned a Research Fellowship in Thoracic Oncology at Tor Vergata University of Rome with a research on the surgical treatment of lung metastases with stages in worldwide well-known oncologic centers: 1) Royal Brompton Hospital (London) 2) Hopital Marie Lannelongue (Paris), 3) Toronto General Hospital (Toronto), 4) MD Anderson Cancer Center (Houston).

In 2000 he was enrolled as Assistant Professor at the Department of Thoracic Surgery directed by Prof. Tommaso Claudio Mineo at the University of Rome Tor Vergata hosted at the Sant'Eugenio Hospital in Rome. There, he served until 2002 when he moved at the new Polyclinic of the Tor Vergata with the task of responsible of the Unit of Thoracic Endoscopy and Videothoracoscopy.

In 2012 he became Associate Professor in Thoracic Surgery at the Department of Experimental Medicine and Surgery of the University of Rome - Tor Vergata Polyclinic, where he is presently carrying out his clinical activities.

Professional Appointments: Policlinico Tor Vergata University, Via Oxford, 81, 00133, Rome, Italy

Publications from the Last 3 Years:

1. Ambrogi V, Tacconi F, Verzicco R. You were not made to live like brutes, but to follow virtue and knowledge. *Ann Thorac Surg.* 2021 Apr 8:S0003-4975(21)00667-6. doi: 10.1016/j.athoracsur.2021.03.086. Epub ahead of print. PMID: 33839131.
2. Vanni G, Materazzo M, Pellicciaro M, Amir S, Tacconi F, Ambrogi V, Buonomo OC. Breast Textured Implants Determine Early T-helper Impairment: BIAL2.20 Study. *Anticancer Res.* 2021 Apr;41(4):2123-2132. doi: 10.21873/anticanres.14984. PMID: 33813423.

3. Tacconi F, Chegai F, Perretta T, Ambrogi V. Real-Time Pleural Elastography: Potential Usefulness in Nonintubated Video-Assisted Thoracic Surgery. *J Chest Surg.* 2021 Jan 21. doi: 10.5090/kjtcs.20.121. Epub ahead of print. PMID: 33767023.
4. Ambrogi V, La Rocca E, Carlea F, Tacconi F. Off label use of T-Tube as chest drainage for uniportal surgery. *Ann Thorac Surg.* 2021 Mar 5:S0003-4975(21)00441-0. doi: 10.1016/j.athoracsur.2021.01.075. Epub ahead of print. PMID: 33684347.
5. Ambrogi V, Tacconi F, Sellitri F, Tamburrini A, Perroni G, Carlea F, La Rocca E, Vanni G, Schillaci O, Mineo TC. Subxiphoid completion thymectomy for refractory non-thymomatous myasthenia gravis. *J Thorac Dis.* 2020 May;12(5):2388-2394. doi: 10.21037/jtd.2020.03.81. PMID: 32642144; PMCID: PMC7330301.
6. Ambrogi V. Preface. *Thorac Surg Clin.* 2020 Feb;30(1):xi-xii. doi: 10.1016/j.thorsurg.2019.09.004. PMID: 31761289.
7. Ambrogi V, Tajè R, Mineo TC. Nonintubated Video-Assisted Wedge Resections in Peripheral Lung Cancer. *Thorac Surg Clin.* 2020 Feb;30(1):49-59. doi: 10.1016/j.thorsurg.2019.08.006. PMID: 31761284.
8. Tacconi F, Mineo TC, Ambrogi V. Team Training for Nonintubated Thoracic Surgery. *Thorac Surg Clin.* 2020 Feb;30(1):111-120. doi: 10.1016/j.thorsurg.2019.08.010. PMID: 31761279.
9. He J, Liu J, Zhu C, Dai T, Cai K, Zhang Z, Cheng C, Qiao K, Liu X, Wang G, Xu S, Yang R, Fan J, Li H, Jin J, Dong Q, Liang L, Ding J, He K, Liu Y, Ye J, Feng S, Jiang Y, Huang H, Zhang H, Liu Z, Feng X, Xia Z, Ma M, Duan Z, Huang T, Li Y, Shen Q, Tan W, Ma H, Sun Y, Chen C, Cui F, Wang W, Li J, Hao Z, Liu H, Liang W, Zou X, Liang H, Yang H, Li Y, Jiang S, Ng CSH, González-Rivas D, Pompeo E, Flores RM, Shargall Y, Ismail M, Ambrogi V, Elkhouly AG, Sung SW, Ang K. Expert consensus on tubeless video-assisted thoracoscopic surgery (Guangzhou). *J Thorac Dis.* 2019 Oct;11(10):4101-4108. doi: 10.21037/jtd.2019.10.04. PMID: 31737292; PMCID: PMC6837991.

10. Vanni G, Materazzo M, Perretta T, Meucci R, Anemona L, Buonomo C, Dauri M, Granai AV, Rho M, Ingallinella S, Tacconi F, Ambrogi V, Chiaravalloti A, Schillaci O, Petrella G, Buonomo OC. Impact of Awake Breast Cancer Surgery on Postoperative Lymphocyte Responses. *In Vivo*. 2019 Nov-Dec;33(6):1879-1884. doi: 10.21873/invivo.11681. PMID: 31662515; PMCID: PMC6899130.
11. Mineo TC, Ambrogi V. Surgical Techniques for Myasthenia Gravis: Video-Assisted Thoracic Surgery. *Thorac Surg Clin*. 2019 May;29(2):165-175. doi: 10.1016/j.thorsurg.2018.12.005. Epub 2019 Mar 7. PMID: 30927998.
12. Zagoriti Z, Lagoumintzis G, Perroni G, Papathanasiou G, Papadakis A, Ambrogi V, Mineo TC, Tzartos JS, Poulas K. Evidence for association of STAT4 and IL12RB2 variants with Myasthenia gravis susceptibility: What is the effect on gene expression in thymus? *J Neuroimmunol*. 2018 Jun 15;319:93-99. doi: 10.1016/j.jneuroim. 2018.03.008. Epub 2018 Mar 17. PMID: 29576322.

In: Mesothelioma
Editor: Albert K. Martin

ISBN: 978-1-68507-075-5
© 2021 Nova Science Publishers, Inc.

Chapter 4

NEW DEVELOPMENTS IN MESOTHELIOMA MARKERS

Gregorio Bonsignore[1], Simona Martinotti[1,2], Federica Grosso[3,4] and Elia Ranzato[1,2],*

[1]University of Piemonte Orientale,
DiSIT - Dipartimento di Scienze e Innovazione Tecnologica,
Alessandria, Italy

[2]University of Piemonte Orientale,
DiSIT - Dipartimento di Scienze e Innovazione Tecnologica,
Vercelli, Italy

[3]Mesothelioma and Rare Cancer Unit,
Azienda Ospedaliera SS Antonio e Biagio e Cesare Arrigo,
Alessandria, Italy

[4]Translational Medicine Unit,
Dipartimento Attività Integrate Ricerca e Innovazione (DAIRI),
Azienda Ospedaliera SS Antonio e Biagio e Cesare Arrigo,
Alessandria, Italy

* Corresponding Author's E-mail: elia.ranzato@uniupo.it.

ABSTRACT

Malignant mesothelioma is a rare cancer arising from serosal surface of the body. Its incidence is strictly related to asbestos exposure, that confers a long-term risk of developing this cancer.

So, due to poor therapy options and long latency time for exposure, there is an urgent need to explore new markers for mesothelioma diagnosis and treatment follow-up.

In this chapter, we will explore the main cancer markers utilized for mesothelioma diagnosis as well as the new developments in the field.

Keywords: biomarkers, malignant mesothelioma

INTRODUCTION

Malignant Mesothelioma

Malignant mesothelioma is a rare but fatal disease, it comes from mesothelial cells and it can hit all serosa (Alpert, van Gerwen, and Taioli 2020). Whereas the data provided by VI report Renam/Inail 2018, 90% of malignant mesothelioma affects pleura, 6,5% peritoneum, 0,003% pericardium and only 0,002% vagina and testis (Bibby et al. 2016).

World Health Organization defines three subtypes of mesothelioma: epithelioid which has a better prognosis, biphasic (intermediate) and sarcomatous which is the worst (Grosso et al. 2016). There are other forms of mesothelioma, they are called borderline: multicystic mesothelioma (more common in woman) and papillary mesothelioma, this latter is very rare but it could shift into epithelioid mesothelioma (Bonadonna, Robustelli della Cuna, and Valagussa 2009; Taddei et al. 2018).

It was demonstrated (Riva et al. 2010) correlation between asbestos and that disease (Yang, Testa, and Carbone 2008; McDonald and McDonald 1996). After exposure to asbestos, mesothelioma has a period of latency, on average 30 years. The mortality rate is very high, and the disease can last about 9-12 months (Bonadonna, Robustelli della Cuna, and Valagussa 2009; Yang, Testa, and Carbone 2008).

Every year mesothelioma kills about 107.000 people, it is rare for young people but its rate increases among middle-aged people (Alpert, van Gerwen, and Taioli 2020).

Asbestos

The term "Asbestos" is used to identify a category of fibres, in this group there are inosilicates and phyllosilicates. According to International Agency for Research on Cancer (IARC) asbestos includes two categories:

- Amphiboles: Actinolite, Grunerite, Anthophyllite, Crocidolite and Tremolite;
- Chrysotile (white asbestos).

These categories have different effect, for example crocidolite and tremolite are more carcinogenic than Chrysotile (Hillerdal 1999).

Small fibres (length exceeding 5 µm and length/width ratio 3:1) are the most dangerous because they can get to the lungs easily. Only one asbestos fibre can't cause mesothelioma, it need a cumulative dose (Iwatsubo et al. 1998).

The asbestos mining started in XX century, it was used in many fields: thermal insulation, textile industry, construction, transport sector.

The discovery of carcinogenic effects has caused very strong reactions by many countries. However, in some regions, asbestos is still used for water disinfection (Crivellari et al. 2015; Hillerdal 1999; Bonadonna, Robustelli della Cuna, and Valagussa 2009).

Professional exposition is not the only way to develop malignant mesothelioma, a proof of that is given by the families of workers. In fact, unfortunately, asbestos fibres can become attached to clothes and hairs, this condition allow them to reach other people (Hillerdal 1999).

Cancer Markers

Cancer markers, or biomarkers, are very different compounds with a specific molecular structure, they normally have a low concentration but could increase in case of cancer. Among them, there are oligoelement (Ca, Cu, Zn), antigens, immunological antibodies, normal proteins (ferritin and thyroglobulin), enzymes (phosphatase), hormones (ectopic hormones), metabolites (polyamine) (Comandone; Correale, Paradiso, and Quaranta 2002a; Holdenrieder et al. 2016; Nathaniel 1981).

Recently, new cancer markers were discovered, as a result, we have a new definition of them:

- substances released by the tumour (directly or indirectly), they could be used to differentiate the tumour from normal tissue or to identify a tumour through the analysis of bodily fluid (blood, urine, saliva, cerebrospinal fluid) produced by the tissues.
- alterations of molecules, processes or substances in cancerous or pre-cancerous conditions. These variations can be founded by specific tests.

Biochemical Indicators Linked to Cancer Development

To be a good cancer marker, it should indicate the extension of disease and its clinic and biologic behaviour, moreover, it should be measurable, standardised, reproducible and expressed only in malignant lesions. In addition, a good cancer marker should have high sensibility to quickly identify cancer cells (before clinic symptoms) and high specificity to allow a specific diagnosis (Duffy 2013; Gion et al. 2011).

There are five type of cancer markers: early indicators, diagnostic factors, prognostic factors, predictive factors and therapeutic targets (Bonadonna, Robustelli della Cuna, and Valagussa 2009).

Early diagnosis allow to find a cancer during preclinical phase (period of time between the appearance and the manifestation of disease)(Correale,

Paradiso, and Quaranta 2002b). Early cancer markers are very useful during this phase; they give information about risk to develop cancer or to individuate tumour in early phase.

For these reasons, they allow to increase or decrease hunch of future neoplastic diseases for patients (Hayes et al. 1996; Sturgeon et al. 2008). Early cancer markers are only used to diagnosticate diseases with high incidence, known prognosis and treatment (Schrohl et al. 2003).

Patients with advanced cancer are very difficult to treat, for this reason early detection is essential. As a result, science community found other markers (Correale, Paradiso, and Quaranta 2002b).

Histopathological diagnosis is the most important example of cancer marker. After the biopsy, diagnostical factors allow to distinguish malignant tissues from benign tissues. Moreover, markers give information about tumour extension and histologic subtype. However, diagnosis cannot be based only on cancer markers because they are not specific, therefore, they could be used with other clinic and experimental exams (Correale, Paradiso, and Quaranta 2002b; Duffy 2013; Hayes et al. 1996).

Cancer markers are commonly used to monitor neoplastic diseases, because of that they are called prognostic factors. Since prognosis gives a forecast of survival ratio, it is important quantify prognostic indicators to identify patients with aggressive disease or to distinguish them from people which don't need other therapies (Correale, Paradiso, and Quaranta 2002b; Duffy 2013).

Predictive markers are factors which give information about successful therapies for single patient or small groups, they are analysed and classified to get details about the individual response to drugs or know individual risk to have side effects.

In cancer therapy, accurate predictive markers have an important role because they can lead to the right treatment, it shows that a specific drug could have different effect in patients with the same histologic subtype of malignant tumour (Correale, Paradiso, and Quaranta 2002b; Duffy 2013).

Finally, if a tumoral pattern is considered suitable, biomarkers are classified like therapeutic targets.

Cancer Markers in Malignant Mesothelioma

It is very difficult to distinguish mesothelioma from other neoplastic diseases like carcinoma. In fact, it is hard to discriminate pleural mesothelioma from peripheric adenocarcinoma and metastatic adenocarcinoma, as well as it is difficult to distinguish peritoneal mesothelioma from papillary peritoneal serous carcinoma and ovarian metastatic serous carcinoma.

Immunochemical Markers

Immunohistochemistry is the most common approach for diagnosing malignant mesothelioma, antigens of cells and tissues are identified by specific antibodies combined with fluorescent or enzymatic tracers. A combination of most frequent markers in mesothelioma (positive markers), carcinoma and sarcoma (negative markers) are used in this approach.

The most relevant positive markers are calretinin, CK 5/6, WT1, D2-40, podoplanin and thrombomorphin.

Calretinin is the most sensitive (95%) and specific (87%) marker. It is positive both in normal and in tumoral mesothelial cells with different cytoplasmic marking (Chhieng et al. 2000).

Antobodies anti-CK 5/6 are useful to differentiate malignant mesotheliomas from pulmonary adenocarcinoma and sarcoma (Shield and Koivurinne 2008).

WT1 (tumour protein Wilms-1) is a marker which was newly included in the guidelines for mesothelioma differential diagnosis. A recent interest focused on sensitivity and specificity of anti-WT1 to distinguish epithelioid mesothelioma from pulmonary adenocarcinoma (Chapel et al. 2020).

D2-40 is a monoclonal antibody which reacts with a 40 kDa antigen, called oncofoetal M2A, in tumoral germinal cells. Recently, immunostaining for D2-40 is more present in mesothelioma than in carcinoma and, for this reason, it should be used to distinguish them (Ordóñez 2005).

Podoplanin is a membrane mucoprotein, it was discovered in rat glomerular endothelial cells. Kimura and colleagues (Kimura and Kimura 2005) reported that, it is more expressed in mesothelioma than in adenocarcinoma, therefore, it's possible to use podoplanin for differential diagnosis.

CD141 was the first marker employed in diagnosis. However, it is expressed in angiosarcoma and squamous carcinoma. For this reason, it is replaced with other markers.

The best known, negative markers are MOC-31, CD15 (Leu-M1), Ber-EP4, CEA and B72.3.

MOC-31 is a monoclonal antibody; it can identify an adhesion molecule on epithelial cells called Ep-CAM. It is considered one of most sensitive and specific negative markers of mesothelioma. Immunostaining for MOC-31 is positive in carcinomas but almost never in mesothelioma tissues (Chapel et al. 2020).

Ber-EP4, an antibody to EpCAM (epithelial cell adhesion molecule), is used to rule out pleural or peritoneal mesothelioma, because it can identify only pulmonary adenocarcinoma and serous carcinoma. Latza et al. (Latza et al. 1990) have shown that Ber-EP4 reacts in 99% of cases with carcinoma but in 0% with mesothelioma.

CEA (carcinoembryonic antigen) is a glycoprotein produced during foetal development and involved in cellular adhesion. CEA is very specific and sensitive and, for this reason, it is counted among the best negative markers to distinguish pulmonary adenocarcinoma from epithelioid mesothelioma.

B72.3 is a monoclonal antibody which reacts against TAG-72, a tumour associated protein. The latter is expressed in many cancers, except in epithelioid mesothelioma (Ordóñez 2005; Combaz-Liar 2015).

Genetic Markers

A genetic marker is a nucleotides sequence and it must have these features:

- polymorphism: the marker must have at least two alternative alleles, the rarest of these must be found in 1% of population (at least);
- mendelian segregation;
- stability across generations,
- easy identification.

Common somatic mutations, in malignant mesothelioma, are recognized in the following genes:

- CDK2NA which gives information about p16
- NF2 which encodes for Merlin protein
- BAP1 which is linked with a protein involved in genetic recombination (DNA repair system).

These genetic variations make a complex individual genetic pattern, probably linked with malignant mesothelioma development; as a result, these genes are considered as markers of mesothelioma (Bott et al. 2011; Grosso et al. 2015).

CDK2NA is one of the main drivers of carcinogenicity, it seems to be involved in hereditary predisposition for malignant mesothelioma. CDK2NA is mutated or down-regulated in many tumoral diseases, therefore, p16 loses its principal functions: CDK (cyclin dependant kinase) inhibition and cell cycle inhibition

There is an epigenetic mutation in 70% of mesothelioma patients, it is caused by a deletion on CDK2NA (Sarun et al. 2018).

The loss of CDK2NA and p16 is useful for differential diagnosis, because it allows to distinguish mesothelioma from other proliferations and found sarcomatous component of it (Betti et al. 2015; Combaz-Liar 2015; Stahel et al. 2015).

If it is inactivated by mutation or deletion, another gene, called NF2, is involved in mesothelioma development. It is located on the short arm of the 22q11 chromosome, which codifies for Neurofibromin 2 (or Merlin). This protein is associated to cytoskeleton, it is involved in cellular motility and communication; in addition, it has an important role in different pathways of signalling, for example NF2/Hippo. In mesothelioma patients, inactivation of NF2 determines the interruption of NF2/Hippo pathway, which causes an alteration of microtubules.

Actually, a direct association between NF2 expression and mesothelioma specific histologic subtypes is not identified; however, supplementary investigations of Merlin protein should lead to new and attractive treatment approaches (Combaz-Liar 2015; Poulikakos et al. 2006; Scagliotti et al. 2018; Stahel et al. 2015).

Another tumour-suppressor gene, commonly altered in malignant mesothelioma and recently identified, is BAP1. Genomic analysis show, that there are BAP1 mutations in 21% of mesothelioma patients, mutations can be missense, nonsense or frameshift. Gene is located on locus 3p21 and it codifies for a nuclear protein which has deubiquitinating role and it's involved in many cellular processes like proliferation and DNA repair. Immunohistochemistry analysis have shown that, BAP1 inactivation is more common in epithelioid mesothelioma than in other subtypes. This result should help for differential diagnosis, but above all for identification of people with high level risk for mesothelioma. These findings should allow to operate patients during the early phase of the disease (Combaz-Liar 2015; Grosso et al. 2015; Testa et al. 2011; Scagliotti et al. 2018; Carbone et al. 2013; Carbone et al. 2016; Pastorino et al. 2018).

Soluble Markers of Mesothelioma

The examination of liquid samples, like serum or pleural effusion, is the most innovative approach to find soluble markers. These molecules, should have an important diagnostic and prognostic role in mesothelioma therapy. Among these, fibulin-3, ostheopontin and mesothelin (which has received the approval of the food and drug administration for clinical use) are the most promising (Porcel 2018; Rossini et al. 2018).

Unfortunately, several soluble markers aren't specific and sensitive enough to identify cancer and, for this reason they are still under study (Kovac et al. 2015).

Mesothelin

This molecule has generated a lot of interest among mesothelioma experts. It is a membrane glycoprotein expressed in mesothelial cells around pleura, pericardium and peritoneum. Human mesothelin is synthesized in the form of 69 kDa polypeptide, it has a hydrophobic sequence on the C-term, this chain is then replaced by glycosylphosphatidylinositol. Later, the intracellular protease Furin causes a proteolytic split which leads to the formation of two different proteins:

MPF = Megakaryocyte Potentiating Factor (32 kDa, soluble);

Mesothelin (40 kDa, membrane protein) (Hassan et al. 2006; Sapède-Peroz 2008).

There are not enough informations about mesothelin biological role, but, recent studies have shown an involvement in adhesion, signalling (received/sent) and survival (Iuzzolini 2017; Tang, Qian, and Ho 2013).

Mesothelin is overexpressed in many human cancers, like mesothelioma and ovary carcinoma. There are two most important hypotheses to explain this condition: a splicing error codifies for a protein, which can not stick to the cell membrane; or protein can stick to cell membrane, but, then a protease removes it (Sapède-Peroz 2008).

Because of the selective expression in some cancers, mesothelin is recognized like potential soluble biomarker. It has a 95% specificity and 50% sensitivity at the time of diagnosis (Creaney et al. 2014).

Mesothelin is the most interesting marker in mesothelioma differential diagnosis, because it allows to distinguish sick patients from subjects at risk, that are healthy people exposed at asbestos, patients with asbestos-related benign diseases or pulmonary adenocarcinoma which has a "mesothelioma-like" growth.

Dipalma and coworkers have found a correlation between histologic subtype and amount of mesothelin, that it is more expressed in epithelioid mesothelioma than in other subtypes (Dipalma et al. 2011; Iuzzolini 2017).

Mesothelin is also helpful to observe tumoral progression or to assess the response to treatment; but, since more studies are needed, at present, it can't be used for screening (Dipalma et al. 2011).

Mesothelin, for its features, is very immunogenic, for this reason, it can be a molecular target, some drugs can use it to bind the cell and trigger the immune response.

At present, there are three most important agents under studies which use mesothelin:

- Amatuximab (MORAb 009), a chimeric monoclonal antibody;
- CRS-207, an attenuated carrier from Listeria Monocytogenes;
- SS1P, a recombinant immunotoxin.

Preliminary clinical trials shown that, these approaches, could reduce disease extension and improve patient management (Crivellari et al. 2015).

Fibulin-3

Another important soluble biomarker, which gave promising results, is Fibulin-3. It is an extracellular matrix glycoprotein encoded by EFEMP1 gene on 2p16 chromosome.

During cancer development, Fibulin-3 is located in many body systems where it controls cellular migration and proliferation, sometimes it could have oncogenic or oncosoppressive function (Pei et al. 2017; Zhang and Marmorstein 2010a, 2010b).

In particular, in their work Pass et al. (Pass et al. 2012; Pass and Goparaju 2013) shown high plasma concentration of Fibulin-3 (specificity 94% and sensitivity 100%) and also in pleural effusions (specificity 93% and sensitivity 84%) of patients. These data allow to distinguish healthy people exposed to asbestos from mesothelioma cases (Rossini et al. 2018).

Creaney and collaborators (Creaney et al. 2014), subsequently, clarified Fibulin-3 role in clinical practise. This protein has less diagnostic sensitivity than Mesothelin in plasma and pleural fluid but it is helpful to valuate mesothelioma progression.

Therefore, mesothelin is more suitable than Fibulin-3 for diagnosis but it is the opposite for prognosis (Creaney et al. 2014; Cristaudo et al. 2018; Kovac et al. 2015).

Osteopontin and RANTES

Osteopontin is a glycoprotein expressed by osteoblast which is involved in many different biologic processes, for example cellular migration, cell-matrix interaction and immunologic regulation. Recent serum Osteopontin meta-analysis show 57% sensitivity and 81% specificity, underlining not a clear role in mesothelioma differential diagnosis.

In fact, there are high Osteopontin levels both in mesothelioma and in other tumours (like ovary, lung and breast)(Cristaudo et al. 2018; Porcel 2018; Sapède-Peroz 2008).

RANTES, also called CCL5, is a chemotactic cytokine (or chemokine) produced by many immune or tumoral cells. In inflammation, it plays an important role in allowing leucocytes recruitment into the wounded area. RANTES is considered a tumoral growth factor, because it is associated with metastatic diffusion and angiogenesis. Comar and colleague, in 2014, have shown, for the first time, that RANTES increase is related to asbestos chronic exposition; so, it should be a soluble prognostic biomarker for asbestos-induced diseases, like mesothelioma (M Comar 2012; M. Comar et al. 2014).

NEW BIOMARKERS

In the last few years, mesothelioma research has advanced a lot and therapies have been changed, the study and the understanding of epigenetic variations allowed this. In fact, the study of many different epigenetic profiles in cancer development, including analysis on miRNA and DNA methylation levels, has had such an impact in biomedical field that miRNA and methylated genes could be used for diagnosis, prognosis or therapies.

Immunotherapy is a new opportunity for mesothelioma therapy, this treatment exploits the immune system, however it is not approved yet for therapies (Ceresoli, Bombardieri, and D'Incalci 2019; Micolucci 2016).

Epigenetics and miRNA

Epigenetic mechanisms include two principal procedures: DNA methylation and regulation of gene expression by microRNA (miRNA).

DNA methylation is typically on cytosine in CpG region or "CpG island," they are regulatory sequences 200-2000 bp long located upstream of each gene, here there are many cytosine and guanosine separated by a phosphate group. During DNA methylation a methyl group (CH_3) is added in position 5' on the carboxy-terminal residue of the cytosine ring by action of the enzyme DNA methyltransferase.

It is a physiologic mechanism for suppression of gene transcription, which leads to the shutdown of gene expression, preventing the interaction between transcriptional factors and DNA. If this event did not occur, there could be consequences, for example neoplastic transformation. In fact, variations of DNA methylation levels can contribute to cancer genesis and, in mesothelioma they are considered like modulators of asbestos action on mesothelial cells (Ceresoli, Bombardieri, and D'Incalci 2019; Christensen et al. 2009).

Goto and colleagues, for first, have reported the involvement of DNA methylation in mesothelioma. In their report, they identified three hypermethylated genes in mesothelioma (TMEM30B, KAZALD1 and

MAPKL13) and suggested to use them like markers (Ceresoli, Bombardieri, and D'Incalci 2019; Goto et al. 2009).

miRNA is one of the most fascinating biologic discoveries, revolutionizing cellular biology. These molecules are single strand non-coding RNA, 22 nucleotides long, they play an important role in many pathological and physiological processes, for example: immune response, cell growth, proliferation, metabolism, stress response and diseases (including cancer).

miRNAs are involved in many contexts, regulating gene expression with interactions in sequence-specific way with targets; as result, translation will be inhibited and/or primary transcript will be degraded.

In fact, it's estimated that about 60% of protein-coding genes are miRNA direct target, they form a complementary pair with bases between miRNA 3'UTR and 5' (seed region). However, miRNAs have different biologic effects; they could match with different genes and give different pathological effects (Ceresoli, Bombardieri, and D'Incalci 2019; Micolucci 2016)

Most of miRNA are present intracelluarly, but most of them are present in biological fluids, secreted through different ways (protein complex, micro vesicles, lipoproteins).

Extracellular miRNAs control cell proliferation and differentiation, so they are very important for communication between normal cells and cancer cells in tumoral microenvironment. Therefore, miRNA up-regulation or down-regulation are specifically related to aggressive phenotype of mesothelioma.

For these reasons, miRNAs are potential diagnostic and/or prognostic mesothelioma biomarkers, they are easy to analyse and retrieve (Allegra et al. 2012; Micolucci 2016).

Gee et al. (Gee et al. 2010) described members of mR-200 family like potential biomarkers that could be used to distinguish mesothelioma patients from pulmonary adenocarcinoma cases (Birnie et al. 2017; Gee et al. 2010).

Benjamin and colleagues have shown three kind of miRNA (miR-193-3p, miR-200c, miR-192) which can be used to accurately differentiate mesothelioma from adenocarcinoma and other pleural or pulmonary malignancies (100% sensitivity, 94 specificity) (Benjamin et al. 2010; Birnie et al. 2017).

Moreover, miRNA can be helpful to evaluate mesothelioma progression. miRNA-29c-5p was recently identified as prognostic factor (Birnie et al. 2017).

CONCLUSION

There are only few valid biomarkers for the management of mesothelioma, while many new biomarkers have been identified, but their clinical assays have not been completely assessed.

Cancer markers are highly demanded for cancer identification as well as for the selection of patients for suitable treatment.

Despite the advancements of the last years, mesothelioma clinical treatment is still inadeguate and patient survival is desolately poor, so the development of experimental approaches is strongly needed but it will not be advanced until acceptable biomarker assays are established.

Therefore, in the future, biomarker development panel should be completed in parallel with drug development or with new therapeutic approaches.

REFERENCES

Allegra, A., A. Alonci, S. Campo, G. Penna, A. Petrungaro, D. Gerace, and C. Musolino. 2012. "Circulating microRNAs: new biomarkers in diagnosis, prognosis and treatment of cancer (review)." *Int J Oncol* 41 (6): 1897-912. https://doi.org/10.3892/ijo.2012.1647. https://www.ncbi.nlm.nih.gov/pubmed/23026890.

Alpert, N., M. van Gerwen, and E. Taioli. 2020. "Epidemiology of mesothelioma in the 21." *Transl Lung Cancer Res* 9 (Suppl 1): S28-S38. https://doi.org/10.21037/tlcr.2019.11.11. https://www.ncbi.nlm.nih.gov/pubmed/32206568.

Benjamin, H., D. Lebanony, S. Rosenwald, L. Cohen, H. Gibori, N. Barabash, K. Ashkenazi, E. Goren, E. Meiri, S. Morgenstern, M. Perelman, I. Barshack, Y. Goren, T. B. Edmonston, A. Chajut, R. Aharonov, Z. Bentwich, N. Rosenfeld, and D. Cohen. 2010. "A diagnostic assay based on microRNA expression accurately identifies malignant pleural mesothelioma." *J Mol Diagn* 12 (6): 771-9. https://doi.org/10.2353/jmoldx.2010.090169. https://www.ncbi.nlm.nih.gov/pubmed/20864637.

Betti, M., E. Casalone, D. Ferrante, A. Romanelli, F. Grosso, S. Guarrera, L. Righi, S. Vatrano, G. Pelosi, R. Libener, D. Mirabelli, R. Boldorini, C Casadio, M. Papotti, G. Matullo, C. Magnani, and I. Dianzani. 2015. "Inference on germline BAP1 mutations and asbestos exposure from the analysis of familial and sporadic mesotelioma in a high-risk area; Genes, Chromosomes and Cancer." *Genes, Chromosomes and Cancer*.

Bibby, A. C., S. Tsim, N. Kanellakis, H. Ball, D. C. Talbot, K. G. Blyth, N. A. Maskell, and I. Psallidas. 2016. "Malignant pleural mesothelioma: an update on investigation, diagnosis and treatment." *Eur Respir Rev* 25 (142): 472-486. https://doi.org/10.1183/16000617.0063-2016. https://www.ncbi.nlm.nih.gov/pubmed/27903668.

Birnie, K. A., C. M. Prêle, P. J. Thompson, B. Badrian, and S. E. Mutsaers. 2017. "Targeting microRNA to improve diagnostic and therapeutic approaches for malignant mesothelioma." *Oncotarget* 8 (44): 78193-78207. https://doi.org/10.18632/oncotarget.20409. https://www.ncbi.nlm.nih.gov/pubmed/29100460.

Bonadonna, G., G. Robustelli della Cuna, and P. Valagussa. 2009. *Medicina oncologica*. 993-1004. [*Oncological medicine*]

Bott, M., M. Brevet, B. S. Taylor, S. Shimizu, T. Ito, L. Wang, J. Creaney, R. A. Lake, M. F. Zakowski, B. Reva, C. Sander, R. Delsite, S. Powell, Q. Zhou, R. Shen, A. Olshen, V. Rusch, and M. Ladanyi. 2011. "The nuclear deubiquitinase BAP1 is commonly inactivated by somatic mutations and 3p21.1 losses in malignant pleural mesothelioma." *Nat Genet* 43 (7): 668-72. https://doi.org/10.1038/ng.855. https://www.ncbi.nlm.nih.gov/pubmed/21642991.

Carbone, M., D. Shimizu, A. Napolitano, M. Tanji, H. I. Pass, H. Yang, and S. Pastorino. 2016. "Positive nuclear BAP1 immunostaining helps differentiate non-small cell lung carcinomas from malignant mesothelioma." *Oncotarget* 7 (37): 59314-59321. https://doi.org/10.18632/oncotarget.10653. https://www.ncbi.nlm.nih.gov/pubmed/27447750.

Carbone, M., H. Yang, H. I. Pass, T. Krausz, J. R. Testa, and G. Gaudino. 2013. "BAP1 and cancer." *Nat Rev Cancer* 13 (3): 153-9. https://doi.org/10.1038/nrc3459. https://www.ncbi.nlm.nih.gov/pubmed/23550303.

Ceresoli, L., E. Bombardieri, and M. D'Incalci. 2019. "Mesothelioma." *From Research to clinical Practise*: 69-89.

Chapel, D. B., J. J. Schulte, A. N. Husain, and T. Krausz. 2020. "Application of immunohistochemistry in diagnosis and management of malignant mesothelioma." *Transl Lung Cancer Res* 9 (Suppl 1): S3-S27. https://doi.org/10.21037/tlcr.2019.11.29. https://www.ncbi.nlm.nih.gov/pubmed/32206567.

Chhieng, D. C., H. Yee, D. Schaefer, J. F. Cangiarella, J. Jagirdar, L. A. Chiriboga, and J. M. Cohen. 2000. "Calretinin staining pattern aids in the differentiation of mesothelioma from adenocarcinoma in serous effusions." *Cancer* 90 (3): 194-200. https://doi.org/10.1002/1097-0142(20000625)90:3<194::aid-cncr8>3.0.co;2-k. https://www.ncbi.nlm.nih.gov/pubmed/10896333.

Christensen, B. C., E. A. Houseman, J. J. Godleski, C. J. Marsit, J. L. Longacker, C. R. Roelofs, M. R. Karagas, M. R. Wrensch, R. F. Yeh, H. H. Nelson, J. L. Wiemels, S. Zheng, J. K. Wiencke, R. Bueno, D. J. Sugarbaker, and K. T. Kelsey. 2009. "Epigenetic profiles distinguish pleural mesothelioma from normal pleura and predict lung asbestos burden and clinical outcome." *Cancer Res* 69 (1): 227-34. https://doi.org/10. 1158/0008-5472.CAN-08-2586. https://www.ncbi.nlm.nih.gov/pubmed/19118007.

Comandone, A. "I marcatori tumorali: vecchi esami per una patologia in evoluzione." *Rete oncologica Piemonte - Valle d'Aosta*: 2-49. ["Tumor markers: old tests for an evolving pathology." *Piedmont Oncology Network - Aosta Valley*]

Comar, M. 2012. *Nuovi marcatori bioumorali nella diagnosi precoce di patologie asbesto correlate.* [*New biohumoral markers in the early diagnosis of asbestos-related diseases*]

Comar, M., N. Zanotta, A. Bonotti, M. Tognon, C. Negro, A. Cristaudo, and M. Bovenzi. 2014. "Increased levels of C-C chemokine RANTES in asbestos exposed workers and in malignant mesothelioma patients from an hyperendemic area." *PLoS One* 9 (8): e104848. https://doi.org/10.1371/journal.pone.0104848. https://www.ncbi.nlm.nih.gov/pubmed/25162674.

Combaz-Liar, C. 2015. "Aspects cliniques et histopathologiques du mésothéliome pleural malin chez l'enfant et l'adulte jeune: à propos d'une série de 47 cas." *Médecine humaine et pathologie*: 1-120. ["Clinical and Histopathological Aspects of Malignant Pleural Mesothelioma in Children and Young Adults: A Report on a Series of 47 Cases." *Human medicine and pathology*]

Correale, M., A. Paradiso, and M. Quaranta. 2002a. "I Markers tumorali: storia, applicazioni e prospettive." *Caleidoscopio*: 5-4. ["Tumor Markers: History, Applications and Perspectives." *Kaleidoscope*]

---. 2002b. "I Markers tumorali: storia, applicazioni e prospettive." *Caleidoscopio*: 5-49. ["Tumor Markers: History, Applications and Perspectives." *Kaleidoscope*]

Creaney, J., I. M. Dick, T. M. Meniawy, S. L. Leong, J. S. Leon, Y. Demelker, A. Segal, A. W. Musk, Y. C. Lee, S. J. Skates, A. K. Nowak, and B. W. Robinson. 2014. "Comparison of fibulin-3 and mesothelin as markers in malignant mesothelioma." *Thorax* 69 (10): 895-902. https://doi.org/10.1136/thoraxjnl-2014-205205. https://www.ncbi.nlm.nih.gov/pubmed/25037982.

Cristaudo, A., A. Bonotti, G. Guglielmi, P. Fallahi, and R. Foddis. 2018. "Serum mesothelin and other biomarkers: what have we learned in the last decade?" *J Thorac Dis* 10 (Suppl 2): S353-S359. https://doi.org/

10.21037/jtd.2017.10.132. https://www.ncbi.nlm.nih.gov/pubmed/29507805.

Crivellari, S., G. Galizzi, F. Ugo, D. Degiovanni, and F. Grosso. 2015. "Il paradosso amianto: il suo utilizzo, la sua diffusione e le sue implicazioni nello sviluppo delle patologie asbesto-correlate." *Working Paper of Public Health* (4(1)): 3-8. ["The asbestos paradox: its use, its spread and its implications in the development of asbestos-related diseases."]

Dipalma, N., V. Luisi, F. Di Serio, A. Fontana, P. Maggiolini, B. Licchelli, E. Mera, L. Bisceglia, I. Galise, M. Loizzi, M. A. Pizzigallo, R. Molinini, and L. Vimercati. 2011. "Biomarkers in malignant mesothelioma: diagnostic and prognostic role of soluble mesothelin-related peptide." *Int J Biol Markers* 26 (3): 160-5. https://doi.org/10.5301/JBM.2011.8614. https://www.ncbi.nlm.nih.gov/pubmed/21928246.

Duffy, M. J. 2013. "Tumor markers in clinical practice: a review focusing on common solid cancers." *Med Princ Pract* 22 (1): 4-11. https://doi.org/10.1159/000338393. https://www.ncbi.nlm.nih.gov/pubmed/22584792.

Gee, G. V., D. C. Koestler, B. C. Christensen, D. J. Sugarbaker, D. Ugolini, G. P. Ivaldi, M. B. Resnick, E. A. Houseman, K. T. Kelsey, and C. J. Marsit. 2010. "Downregulated microRNAs in the differential diagnosis of malignant pleural mesothelioma." *Int J Cancer* 127 (12): 2859-69. https://doi.org/10.1002/ijc.25285. https://www.ncbi.nlm.nih.gov/pubmed/21351265.

Gion, M., C. Trevisol, S. Pregno, and A. S. C. Fabricio. 2011. Guida all'uso clinico dei biomarcatori in oncologia: premesse e generalità; *Biochimica Clinica*. (35(2)): 97-106. [Guide to the clinical use of biomarkers in oncology: background and general information; *Clinical Biochemistry*.]

Goto, Y., K. Shinjo, Y. Kondo, L. Shen, M. Toyota, H. Suzuki, W. Gao, B. An, M. Fujii, H. Murakami, H. Osada, T. Taniguchi, N. Usami, M. Kondo, Y. Hasegawa, K. Shimokata, K. Matsuo, T. Hida, N. Fujimoto, T. Kishimoto, J. P. Issa, and Y. Sekido. 2009. "Epigenetic profiles distinguish malignant pleural mesothelioma from lung adenocarcinoma." *Cancer Res* 69 (23): 9073-82. https://doi.org/10.1158/0008-5472.CAN-09-1595. https://www.ncbi.nlm.nih.gov/pubmed/19887624.

Grosso, F., A. Kasa, G. Galizzi, S. Crivellari, D. Degiovanni, E. Ponte, and S. Zai. 2016. "Il mesotelioma pleurico maligno nel paziente anziano. Studio retrospettivo nei centri di Alessandria e Casale Monferrato." *Working Paper of Public Health* 11 (5(1)): 1-17. ["Malignant pleural mesothelioma in the elderly patient. Retrospective study in the centers of Alessandria and Casale Monferrato."]

Grosso, F., R. Libener, A. Roveta, L. Randi, F. Ugo, M. Bertolotti, M. D'angelo, D. Degiovanni, and G. Ferretti. 2015. "Novità sul trattamento del mesotelioma pleurico maligno." *Working Paper of Public Health* (4(1)): 1-1. ["News on the treatment of malignant pleural mesothelioma."]

Hassan, R., A. T. Remaley, M. L. Sampson, J. Zhang, D. D. Cox, J. Pingpank, R. Alexander, M. Willingham, I. Pastan, and M. Onda. 2006. "Detection and quantitation of serum mesothelin, a tumor marker for patients with mesothelioma and ovarian cancer." *Clin Cancer Res* 12 (2): 447-53. https://doi.org/10.1158/1078-0432.CCR-05-1477. https://www.ncbi.nlm.nih.gov/pubmed/16428485.

Hayes, D. F., R. C. Bast, C. E. Desch, H. Fritsche, N. E. Kemeny, J. M. Jessup, G. Y. Locker, J. S. Macdonald, R. G. Mennel, L. Norton, P. Ravdin, S. Taube, and R. J. Winn. 1996. "Tumor marker utility grading system: a framework to evaluate clinical utility of tumor markers." *J Natl Cancer Inst* 88 (20): 1456-66. https://doi.org/10.1093/jnci/88.20.1456. https://www.ncbi.nlm.nih.gov/pubmed/8841020.

Hillerdal, G. 1999. "Mesothelioma: cases associated with non-occupational and low dose exposures." *Occup Environ Med* 56 (8): 505-13. https://doi.org/10.1136/oem.56.8.505. https://www.ncbi.nlm.nih.gov/pubmed/10492646.

Holdenrieder, S., L. Pagliaro, D. Morgenstern, and F. Dayyani. 2016. "Clinically Meaningful Use of Blood Tumor Markers in Oncology."

Biomed Res Int 2016: 9795269. https://doi.org/10.1155/2016/9795269. https://www.ncbi.nlm.nih.gov/pubmed/28042579.

Iuzzolini, M. 2017. *Valutazione di dosaggi seriati di mesotelina sierica in pazienti affetti da mesotelioma maligno della pleura.* [*Evaluation of serial dosages of serum mesothelin in patients with malignant mesothelioma of the pleura.*]

Iwatsubo, Y., J. C. Pairon, C. Boutin, O. Ménard, N. Massin, D. Caillaud, E. Orlowski, F. Galateau-Salle, J. Bignon, and P. Brochard. 1998. "Pleural mesothelioma: dose-response relation at low levels of asbestos exposure in a French population-based case-control study." *Am J Epidemiol* 148 (2): 133-42. https://doi.org/10.1093/oxfordjournals.aje.a009616. https://www.ncbi.nlm.nih.gov/pubmed/9676694.

Kimura, N., and I. Kimura. 2005. "Podoplanin as a marker for mesothelioma." *Pathol Int* 55 (2): 83-6. https://doi.org/10.1111/j.1440-1827.2005.01791.x. https://www.ncbi.nlm.nih.gov/pubmed/15693854.

Kovac, V., M. Dodic-Fikfak, N. Arneric, V. Dolzan, and A. Franko. 2015. "Fibulin-3 as a biomarker of response to treatment in malignant mesothelioma." *Radiol Oncol* 49 (3): 279-85. https://doi.org/10.1515/raon-2015-0019. https://www.ncbi.nlm.nih.gov/pubmed/26401134.

Latza, U., G. Niedobitek, R. Schwarting, H. Nekarda, and H. Stein. 1990. "Ber-EP4: new monoclonal antibody which distinguishes epithelia from mesothelial." *J Clin Pathol* 43 (3): 213-9. https://doi.org/10.1136/jcp.43.3.213. https://www.ncbi.nlm.nih.gov/pubmed/1692040.

McDonald, J. C., and A. D. McDonald. 1996. "The epidemiology of mesothelioma in historical context." *Eur Respir J* 9 (9): 1932-42. https://doi.org/10.1183/09031936.96.09091932. https://www.ncbi.nlm.nih.gov/pubmed/8880114.

Micolucci, L. 2016. *Ruolo dei microRNA nella patogenesi del mesotelioma maligno: un approccio basato sulle "evidenze scientifiche" e sull'analisi computazionale.* [*Role of microRNAs in the pathogenesis of malignant mesothelioma: an approach based on "scientific evidence" and computational analysis*]

Nathaniel, I. 1981. "Tumor Markers in Cancer Prevention and Detection." *Cancer*: 1151-1153.

Ordóñez, N. G. 2005. "Immunohistochemical diagnosis of epithelioid mesothelioma: an update." *Arch Pathol Lab Med* 129 (11): 1407-14. https://doi.org/10.1043/1543-2165(2005)129[1407:IDOEMA] 2.0.CO;2. https://www.ncbi.nlm.nih.gov/pubmed/16253021.

Pass, H. I., and C. Goparaju. 2013. "Fibulin-3 as a biomarker for pleural mesothelioma." *N Engl J Med* 368 (2): 190. https://doi.org/10.1056/ NEJMc1213514. https://www.ncbi.nlm.nih.gov/pubmed/23301743.

Pass, H. I., S. M. Levin, M. R. Harbut, J. Melamed, L. Chiriboga, J. Donington, M. Huflejt, M. Carbone, D. Chia, L. Goodglick, G. E. Goodman, M. D. Thornquist, G. Liu, M. de Perrot, M. S. Tsao, and C. Goparaju. 2012. "Fibulin-3 as a blood and effusion biomarker for pleural mesothelioma." *N Engl J Med* 367 (15): 1417-27. https:// doi.org/10.1056/NEJMoa1115050. https://www.ncbi.nlm.nih.gov/pub med/23050525.

Pastorino, S., Y. Yoshikawa, H. I. Pass, M. Emi, M. Nasu, I. Pagano, Y. Takinishi, R. Yamamoto, M. Minaai, T. Hashimoto-Tamaoki, M. Ohmuraya, K. Goto, C. Goparaju, K. Y. Sarin, M. Tanji, A. Bononi, A. Napolitano, G. Gaudino, M. Hesdorffer, H. Yang, and M. Carbone. 2018. "A Subset of Mesotheliomas with Improved Survival Occurring in Carriers of BAP1 and Other Germline Mutations." *J Clin Oncol*: JCO2018790352. https://doi.org/10.1200/JCO.2018.79.0352. https://www.ncbi.nlm.nih.gov/pubmed/30376426.

Pei, D., Y. Li, X. Liu, S. Yan, X. Guo, and X. Xu. 2017. "Diagnostic and prognostic utilities of humoral fibulin-3 in malignant pleural mesothelioma: Evidence from a meta-analysis." *Oncotarget* 8 (8): 13030-13038. https://doi.org/10.18632/oncotarget.14712 https://www.ncbi.nlm.nih.gov/pubmed/28103581.

Porcel, J. M. 2018. "Biomarkers in the diagnosis of pleural diseases: a 2018 update." *Ther Adv Respir Dis* 12: 1753466618808660. https:// doi.org/10.1177/1753466618808660. https://www.ncbi.nlm.nih.gov/ pubmed/30354850.

Poulikakos, P. I., G. H. Xiao, R. Gallagher, S. Jablonski, S. C. Jhanwar, and J. R. Testa. 2006. "Re-expression of the tumor suppressor NF2/merlin inhibits invasiveness in mesothelioma cells and negatively regulates FAK." *Oncogene* 25 (44): 5960-8. https://doi.org/10.1038/sj.onc.1209587. https://www.ncbi.nlm.nih.gov/pubmed/16652148.

Riva, M. A., F. Carnevale, V. A. Sironi, G. De Vito, and G. Cesana. 2010. "Mesothelioma and asbestos, fifty years of evidence: Chris Wagner and the contribution of the Italian occupational medicine community." *Med Lav* 101 (6): 409-15. https://www.ncbi.nlm.nih.gov/pubmed/21141345.

Rossini, M., P. Rizzo, I. Bononi, A. Clementz, R. Ferrari, F. Martini, and M. G. Tognon. 2018. "New Perspectives on Diagnosis and Therapy of Malignant Pleural Mesothelioma." *Front Oncol* 8: 91. https://doi.org/10.3389/fonc.2018.00091. https://www.ncbi.nlm.nih.gov/pubmed/29666782.

Sapède-Peroz. 2008. "Développement de marqueurs diagnostiques et d'approches thérapeutiques pour le mésothéliome pleural malin."

Sarun, K. H., K. Lee, M. Williams, C. M. Wright, C. J. Clarke, N. C. Cheng, K. Takahashi, and Y. Y. Cheng. 2018. "Genomic Deletion of." *Int J Mol Sci* 19 (10). https://doi.org/10.3390/ijms19103056. https://www.ncbi.nlm.nih.gov/pubmed/30301262.

Scagliotti, G. V., P. Bironzo, C. Magnani, G. Rossi, A. Veltri, R. Trisolini, G. Rocco, S. Ramella, F. Grosso, and V. A. Marsico. 2018. "Mesotelioma pleurico: linee guida." *Associazione Italiana di Oncologia Medica*: 16. ["Pleural Mesothelioma: Guidelines." *Italian Association of Medical Oncology*]

Schrohl, A. S., M. Holten-Andersen, F. Sweep, M. Schmitt, N. Harbeck, J. Foekens, N. Brünner, and European Organisation for Research and Treatment of Cancer (EORTC) Receptor and Biomarker Group. 2003. "Tumor markers: from laboratory to clinical utility." *Mol Cell Proteomics* 2 (6): 378-87. https://doi.org/10.1074/mcp.R300006-MCP200. https://www.ncbi.nlm.nih.gov/pubmed/12813140.

Shield, P. W., and K. Koivurinne. 2008. "The value of calretinin and cytokeratin 5/6 as markers for mesothelioma in cell block preparations of serous effusions." *Cytopathology* 19 (4): 218-23. https://doi.org/10.1111/j.1365-2303.2007.00482.x. https://www.ncbi.nlm.nih.gov/pubmed/17916095.

Stahel, R. A., W. Weder, E. Felley-Bosco, U. Petrausch, A. Curioni-Fontecedro, I. Schmitt-Opitz, and S. Peters. 2015. "Searching for targets for the systemic therapy of mesothelioma." *Ann Oncol* 26 (8): 1649-60. https://doi.org/10.1093/annonc/mdv101. https://www.ncbi.nlm.nih.gov/pubmed/25722383.

Sturgeon, C. M., B. R. Hoffman, D. W. Chan, S. L. Ch'ng, E. Hammond, D. F. Hayes, L. A. Liotta, E. F. Petricoin, M. Schmitt, O. J. Semmes, G. Söletormos, E. van der Merwe, E. P. Diamandis, and National Academy of Clinical Biochemistry. 2008. "National Academy of Clinical Biochemistry Laboratory Medicine Practice Guidelines for use of tumor markers in clinical practice: quality requirements." *Clin Chem* 54 (8): e1-e10. https://doi.org/10.1373/clinchem.2007.094144. https://www.ncbi.nlm.nih.gov/pubmed/18606634.

Taddei, S., F. Falco, C. Galeone, R. Piro, and N. C. Facciolongo. 2018. "Mesotelioma pleurico maligno." *Mesotelioma pleurico maligno; Rassegna Di Patologia dell'Apparato Respiratorio* (33(5)): 260-270. ["Malignant Pleural Mesothelioma." Malignant pleural mesothelioma; *Review of Pathology of the Respiratory System*]

Tang, Z., M. Qian, and M. Ho. 2013. "The role of mesothelin in tumor progression and targeted therapy." *Anticancer Agents Med Chem* 13 (2): 276-80. https://doi.org/10.2174/1871520611313020014. https://www.ncbi.nlm.nih.gov/pubmed/22721387.

Testa, J. R., M. Cheung, J. Pei, J. E. Below, Y. Tan, E. Sementino, N. J. Cox, A. U. Dogan, H. I. Pass, S. Trusa, M. Hesdorffer, M. Nasu, A. Powers, Z. Rivera, S. Comertpay, M. Tanji, G. Gaudino, H. Yang, and M. Carbone. 2011. "Germline BAP1 mutations predispose to malignant mesothelioma." *Nat Genet* 43 (10): 1022-5. https://doi.org/10.1038/ng.912. https://www.ncbi.nlm.nih.gov/pubmed/21874000.

Yang, G., J. R. Testa, and M. Carbone. 2008. "Mesothelioma Epidemiology, Carcinogenesis and Pathogenesis." *Current Treatment Options Oncology* (9(2-3)): 147-157.

Zhang, Y., and L. Y. Marmorstein. 2010a. *Focus on Molecules: Fibulin-3, Experimental Eye Research*.

---. 2010b. *Focus on Molecules: Fibulin-3, Experimental Eye Research*.

In: Mesothelioma
Editor: Albert K. Martin

ISBN: 978-1-68507-075-5
© 2021 Nova Science Publishers, Inc.

Chapter 5

SURGICAL APPROACHES TO PLEURAL TUMOURS

Elena Prisciandaro[1], MD,
Luca Bertolaccini[1,*], MD, PhD, Lara Girelli[1], MD
and Lorenzo Spaggiari[1,2], MD, PhD

[1]Department of Thoracic Surgery, IEO,
European Institute of Oncology IRCCS, Milan, Italy
[2]Department of Oncology and Hemato-Oncology,
University of Milan, Milan, Italy

ABSTRACT

The pleurae are serous membranes encasing the lungs and may develop benign and malignant neoplasms. Primary pleural tumours may arise in the visceral pleura, the parietal pleura, or both. Benign tumours are usually confined to the pleura, rarely causing infiltration of the surrounding tissues or distant metastases and has a surgical treatment.

---

* Corresponding Author's E-mail: luca.bertolaccini@gmail.com.

The most common one is malignant pleural mesothelioma (MPM). Mesothelioma is a malignant neoplasm that originates from the mesothelia, the lining sheets of the serous cavities: pleura, pericardium, peritoneum and, in men, the tunica vaginalis of the testicles. In more than 90% of cases, mesothelioma has a pleural localisation (MPM). The current standard-of-care treatment of MPM is generally accepted as systemic therapy alone. Surgery could be part of a multimodal treatment plan since it is the only modality that could render a patient without the disease. Selecting patients fit for surgery, determining the optimal operation, and the additional treatments have not yet been established due to the extreme variability of cancer itself related to the variability of the surgical techniques.

The complete macroscopic resection is the objective of surgical treatment. Surgery (open or VATS pleural biopsies) could help achieve an MPM correct diagnosis or palliate (VATS pleurectomy, VATS talc pleurodesis, indwelling pleural drainage placement) symptoms caused by malignant pleural effusions. Every time aggressive surgery is scheduled, it aims to remove all visible disease, increasing survival by decreasing the intrathoracic tumour burden to microscopic levels. Ideally, all MPM patients should be operated on by Thoracic Surgeons with recognised broad experience in MPM management, regularly related to Radiation and Medical Oncology involved in MPM clinical trials.

Even though there is a brand new, improved MPM staging system, the results of surgery for MPM are strongly influenced by other prognosticators not taken by the current staging system (such as subtype of histology). Consequently, at this time it is not possible to determine a common denominator that permits laborious evaluation between surgical series and ultimate establishing which surgical approach and adjuvants are advantageous and in which sequences/circumstances used or combined.

INTRODUCTION

The pleurae are serous membranes encasing the lungs and may develop benign and malignant neoplasms. Primary pleural tumours may arise in the visceral pleura, the parietal pleura, or both (Table 1).

Table 1. Principal histologies of primary pleural tumours

Primary benign tumours of the pleura	Primary malignant tumours of the pleura
Solitary fibrous tumour of the pleura	Malignant pleural mesothelioma
Pleural lipoma	Pleural liposarcoma
Pleural leiomyoma	Pleural leiomyosarcoma
Pleural schwannoma	Pleural hemangiopericytoma
Pleural haemangioma	Pleural haemangioendothelioma
Pleural endothelioma	Pleural lymphoma
	Synovial sarcoma of the pleura
	Pleural angiosarcoma
	Desmoplastic tumour of the pleura

BENIGN TUMOURS

Benign tumours are usually confined to the pleura, rarely causing infiltration of the surrounding tissues or distant metastases. However, they may reach the remarkable size and cause compression and/or dislocation of intrathoracic anatomical structures, leading to severe and life-threatening cardio-respiratory complications. The most frequent histology is the solitary fibrous tumour of the pleura (SFTP), which may occasionally show features of malignancy, with a tendency towards recurrence and metastatic dissemination.

Clinical Presentation

The SFTP is generally asymptomatic and is diagnosed incidentally. Alternatively, it may manifest itself with cough, dyspnoea and/or chest pain.

Diagnosis

The SFTP is often an incidental finding not related to the disorder(s) that prompted the diagnostic investigation. On chest X-ray, the SFTP appears as a sessile or pedunculated opacity originating from in the pleura, sometimes associated with opacification of the ipsilateral costophrenic recess (due to pleural effusion). Computed tomography (CT) of the chest shows a highly vascular mass contiguous to the pleura, homogeneous after injection of contrast enhancement, sometimes with hypodense areas within (necrosis or intratumoral haemorrhages). A definite diagnosis can only be made by histological examination of specimens obtained by transthoracic (tru-cut) or surgical biopsy.

Therapy

The SFTP has a surgical treatment. Radical resection is essential to minimise the risk of local recurrence. First, a careful exploration of the pleural cavity is mandatory to identify pleural effusion (which is then aspirated for cytological examination) and/or previously unknown pleural and pericardial lesions. Then, complete excision of the pleural tumour with resection of any intraparenchymal pulmonary foci by segmentectomy or lobectomy is performed, usually by video-assisted thoracic surgery (VATS). However, in case of large tumour size or infiltration of the chest wall, pericardium and/or diaphragm, a thoracotomy approach is preferred.

MALIGNANT TUMOURS

The most common one is malignant pleural mesothelioma (MPM). Mesothelioma is a malignant neoplasm that originates from the mesothelia, the lining sheets of the serous cavities: pleura, pericardium, peritoneum and, in men, the tunica vaginalis of the testicles. In more than 90% of cases, mesothelioma has a pleural localisation (MPM).

Epidemiology and Aetiology

Exposure to Asbestos

The main risk factor for the onset of MPM is exposure to asbestos, which has been listed among the occupational carcinogens by the World Health Organisation (WHO). The time interval between the beginning of the asbestos exposure and the onset of mesothelioma is highly variable (20-50 years). However, the onset is earlier in individuals who have had more intense exposure to asbestos (dose-dependent effect). As an asbestos-related disease, MPM most frequently affects men aged 60-65 on average.

Three leading causes of asbestos exposure are recognised:

- Environmental exposure: Although it is a rare neoplasm (about 2.2 cases per million inhabitants), MPM reaches unexpected peaks of incidence in built-up areas located near industrial and manufacturing complexes where asbestos was processed (iron and steel, automotive, textile, chemical and petrochemical sectors, shipbuilding, thermoelectric power stations).
- Occupational exposure: workers extracting, separating, handling, carding, spinning and weaving asbestos, insulation workers, railway workers, seafarers, farmers.
- Domestic exposure: due to the presence of asbestos in some commonly used items (stoves, boilers, radiators, hairdryers) and in materials used for building construction.

Asbestos fibres have extremely variable length and thickness, the most harmful being those longer than 5-8 μm and with a diameter of fewer than 0.25 μm, which can reach the periphery of the lung by evading the macrophage and mucociliary elimination systems. The prolonged interaction of asbestos with cellular elements underlies the self-maintaining mechanisms of inflammation: frustrated phagocytosis and oxidative burst generate a vicious cycle that perpetuates the inflammatory response, further damaging the lung parenchyma and pleural serosa. Asbestos interferes with the signalling systems of mesothelial cells at different levels, causing them to mutate and immortalise, leading to the tumour's birth, progression, and neoangiogenesis. The most common cytogenetic alteration found in asbestos-induced mesothelioma is the 9p21 homozygosis deletion, which causes the loss of a cluster of genes including CDKN2A, CDKN2B and MTAP. The oncosuppressor genes CDKN2A and CDKN2B encode for the cell cycle regulatory proteins p14, p15 and p16, while MTAP encodes for a methylthioadenosine phosphorylase. The protein p16 (or INK4a) is an inhibitor of cyclin-dependent kinases (CDKIs), which, in turn, inhibit the antiproliferative activity of the RB protein and allow cell cycle progression. In other words, p16 prevents the G1/S transition: a mutation in it allows the cell to evade the checkpoint systems and assume a neoplastic phenotype, as occurs in many tumours that share a mesodermal origin with mesotheliomas, such as melanoma and renal cell carcinoma.

Other Risk Factors

In 20% of cases, MPM is not asbestos-related. Additional risk factors are:

- Simian Virus 40 (SV40): it is believed that SV40 may act as a co-carcinogen and asbestos, promoting cell proliferation.
- Hereditary factors (BAP-1 cancer syndrome): BAP-1 (BRCA-associated protein 1) is an oncosuppressor gene that promotes DNA damage repair. A mutation can lead to neoplastic transformation and the proliferation of unstable cells. The BAP-1 cancer syndrome is characterised by the association of mesothelioma, uveal melanoma, cutaneous melanoma, MBAIT (atypical intradermal melanocytic tumours) and other neoplasms.
- Exposure to erionite: a fibrous mineral belonging to the zeolite family, which is significantly more carcinogenic and fibrogenic than asbestos.
- Minor risk factors: previous tubercular disease, chronic inflammatory disease, accidental or iatrogenic exposure to ionising

radiation, particularly in individuals who have undergone radiotherapy for breast cancer or mediastinal Hodgkin lymphoma.

Clinical Presentation

The clinical manifestations of MPM are non-specific and appear in the advanced stages of the disease. The onset is characterised by dyspnoea, which may or may not is associated with chest pain. In the early stages, dyspnoea is caused by pleural effusion, which obliterates the costophrenic recess and prevents the lung from expanding. However, in a more advanced stage of disease, it is caused by the pleural thickening incarcerating the lung parenchyma; for this reason, even in the absence of a pleural effusion, ventilation is significantly impaired. Chest pain is unilateral and is often sharp or stabbing. Patients generally locate it in the shoulder, arm, chest wall and/or upper abdomen. It is not responsive to common analgesics, as it is caused by invasion of the chest wall and tends to worsen as the disease progresses. If the thoracic intercostal, autonomic, or brachial nerve plexus is involved, the pain will also have a neuropathic component. Rarely patients complain of cough, asthenia, weight loss, fever, profuse sweating, haemoptysis, or pneumothorax. Expansion of the mass towards the mediastinum may result in dysphagia, phrenic nerve paralysis, pericardial effusion, Horner syndrome or superior vena cava syndrome.

Similarly, the appearance of ascites may indicate the spread of mesothelioma to the peritoneum. The diagnosis of a paraneoplastic syndrome associated with MPM is not uncommon. The most frequent include:

- Thrombocytosis (platelets > 400,000/ml).
- Hypoglycaemic syndrome.
- Pneumonic hypertrophic osteoarthropathy: a form of symmetrical hyperostosis confined to the distal segments of the upper and lower

limbs, causing clubbing associated with pain and functional limitation in the wrists and ankles.

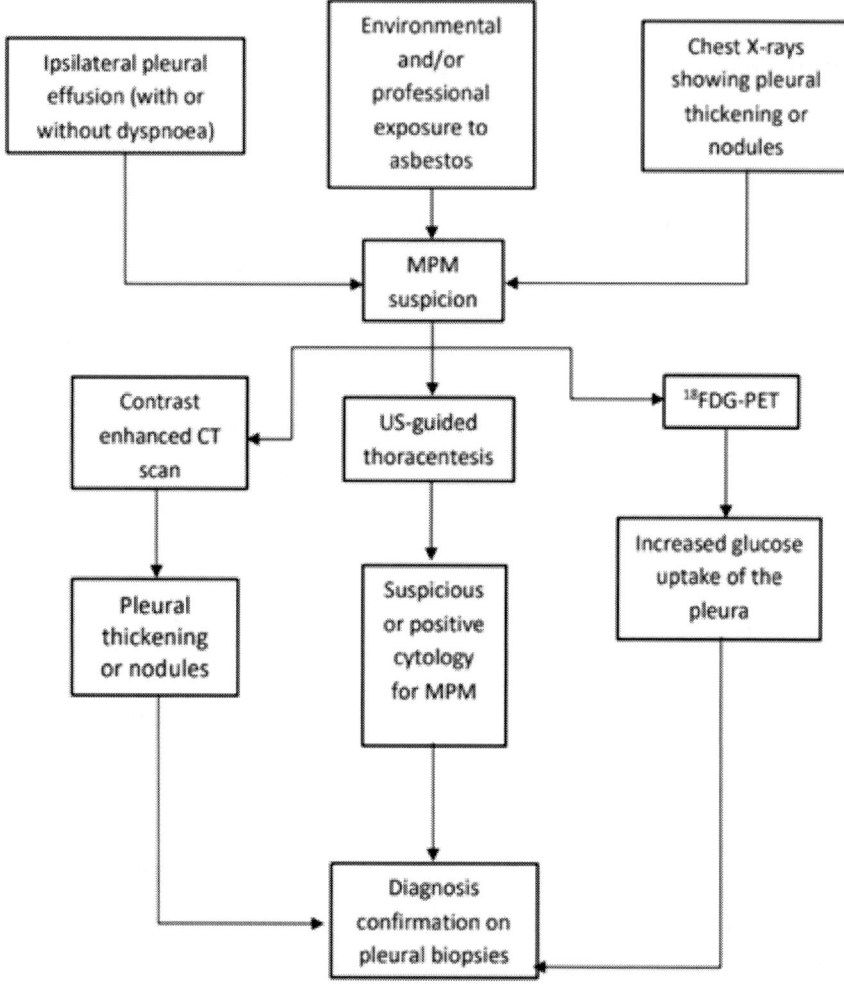

Figure 1. Diagnostic algorithm for MPM.

Diagnosis

The diagnosis of MPM is often delayed, as the disease causes non-specific symptoms and can be attributed to many other diseases. The diagnostic workup includes radiological tests, biochemical and cytological analyses, guided by the patient's history of exposure to asbestos (Figure 1).

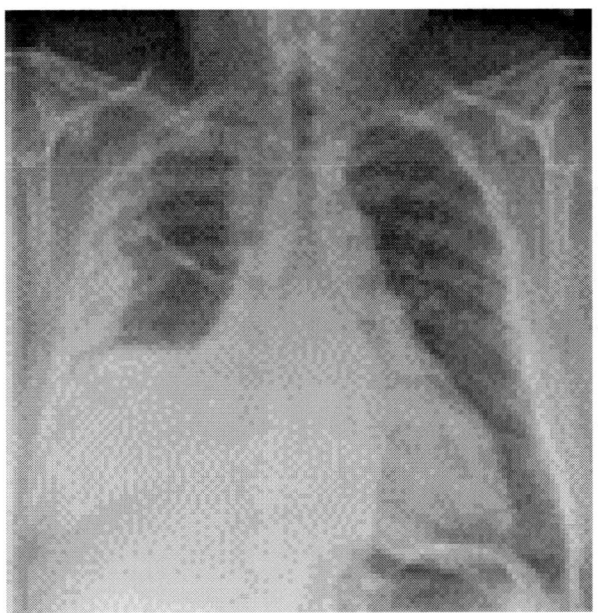

Figure 2. Chest X-ray of a right MPM.

Chest X-Ray

Routinely performed to identify the origin of symptoms, it has low specificity and sensitivity. MPM presents as diffuse unilateral and concentric thickening of the pleura, which may be associated with opacification of the hemithorax starting from the costophrenic recess (from pleural effusion). In the advanced stages of the disease, narrowing the intercostal spaces, elevating the ipsilateral hemidiaphragm, and mediastinal shift ipsilateral to the tumour may appear (Figure 2).

Chest CT Scan with Contrast Enhancement

It provides detailed information on the characteristics of the lesion and the extent of the disease, allowing adequate staging and preoperative management. The most common CT findings include diffuse and irregular pleural thickening or pleural nodularity, sometimes associated with mediastinal nodal disease (Figure 3).

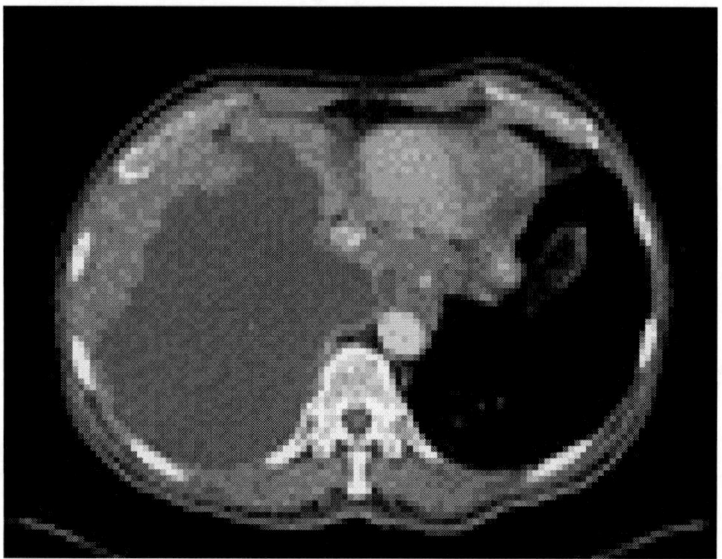

Figure 3. Chest CT scans of a right MPM.

18-Fluorodeoxyglucose Positron Emission Tomography with (18FDG-PET)

It allows increased metabolic activity to be detected in the tissues affected by the neoplasm. It allows detection of possible lymph node involvement and/or the presence of distant metastases.

Magnetic Resonance Imaging (MRI)

It provides a more detailed and in-depth study of the soft tissues than CT, particularly in identifying an isolated focus on the chest wall or invasion of the diaphragm.

Other Radiological Methods

In diagnostic imaging, an ancillary role is reserved for thoracic ultrasounds (US) to perform needle aspiration/biopsy or US-guided drainage.

Tumour Marker Evaluation in Pleural Fluid

Low levels of Carcino-Embryonic Antigen (CEA) and high levels of Tissue Polypeptide Antigen (TPA) and serum Cytokeratin Fragment 21.1 (CYFRA 21.1) in the pleural fluid have been associated with MPM.

Cytological Examination of Pleural Fluid

The reliability and usefulness of cytological analysis of pleural effusion fluid remain the subject of heated debate to date. Although the finding of various cytological abnormalities allows the suspicion of MPM to be raised, cytological examination alone cannot guarantee the certainty of the diagnostic hypothesis.

Pathological Anatomy

Histological examination is performed on surgical bioptic specimens. Morphological and electron microscopy analyses (especially when combined with immunohistochemistry investigations) allow mesothelioma to be identified with almost absolute certainty. The macroscopic appearance of MPM depends on the stage of the disease during which the analysis takes place. Small nodules cover the parietal pleura in the early stages and, less frequently, the visceral pleura. In advanced-stage disease, these nodules tend to coalescence and fuse into a thick and hard rind (Figure 4). The serous cavity is obliterated, and the thickened pleura incarcerates the lung, hindering its physiological expansion (diffuse malignant mesothelioma). Rarely, the tumour may present as a pedunculated or sessile isolated mass (localised malignant mesothelioma) attached to the visceral or parietal pleura. The neoplastic mesothelial tissue differentiates along an epithelial or connective line. The epithelial component has an eosinophilic (acidophilic) and sometimes vacuolated cytoplasm, with round, vesicular, central nuclei, plus a single evident nucleolus. The connective component has intertwined bundles of spindle-shaped cells, markedly pleomorphic (with various morphologies: from round to flattened elements, with little cytoplasm), immersed in a collagenous stroma (Figure 5). Based on the prevalent fraction of neoplastic cells, it is possible to distinguish three main histological types of mesotheliomas:

- Epithelioid, the most frequent variant (60-80% of cases).
- Biphasic or mixed, diagnosed in 10-15% of cases.
- Sarcomatoid or fibrous, accounting for less than 10% of cases.

Fundamental to the mesothelioma diagnosis is determining the tissue immunohistochemical pattern, which is mainly used for the differential diagnosis. Epithelioid MPM must be mainly distinguished from lung adenocarcinoma; to this end, the International Mesothelioma Panel (IMP) suggests the combined use of at least five markers: one generic (such as pancytokeratins and cytokeratins 5/6), two positive (such as calretinin and WT-1) and two negatives (such as TTF-1 and CEA). Immunohistochemistry plays a minor role in the diagnosis of sarcomatoid MPM, as these histotypes only express calretinin, in addition to vimentin and cytokeratin.

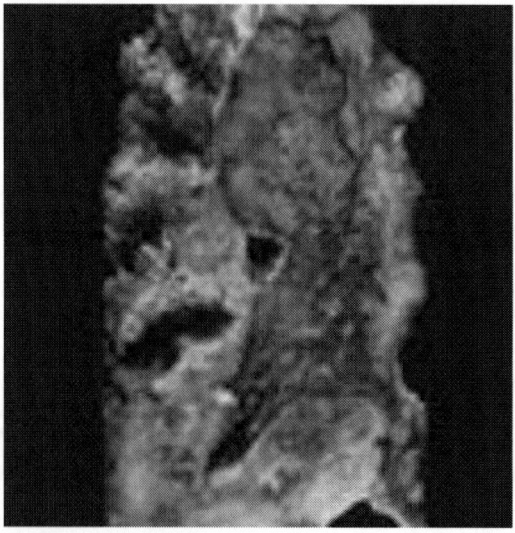

Figure 4. Gross pathology of an MPM.

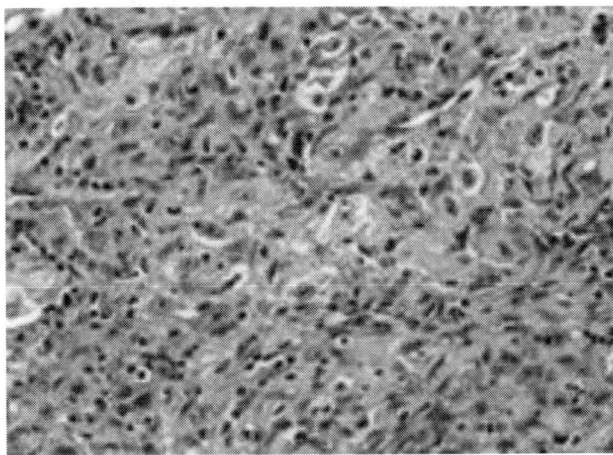

Figure 5. Microscopic pathology of a sarcomatoid MPM.

Prognosis and Staging

MPM needs careful evaluation as it has an inferior prognosis: treatment strategies are currently limited and do not guarantee prolonged disease-free survival. The average life expectancy of patients with MPM is 4-18 months. The prognosis is primarily influenced by the patient's characteristics and general condition, such as:

- Age: younger patients generally have more prolonged survival.
- Gender: men seem to be disadvantaged.
- Performance status, i.e., the ability to carry out everyday activities of daily living.
- Clinical symptoms, such as chest pain or loss of weight and appetite.

The neoplastic histotypes also strongly influence the survival of affected patients: biphasic and sarcomatoid forms have a worse prognosis than epithelioid forms.

Table 2. TNM descriptors

T	
T1	Tumour involving the ipsilateral parietal pleura (including mediastinal and diaphragmatic pleura) without the involvement of visceral pleura
T2	Tumour involving each of the ipsilateral pleural surfaces (parietal, mediastinal, diaphragmatic, and visceral pleura) with at least one of the following features: • A confluent visceral pleural tumour (including the fissures). • Involvement of diaphragmatic muscle). • Invasion of the lung parenchyma
T3	Tumour involving all the ipsilateral pleural surfaces (parietal, mediastinal, diaphragmatic, and visceral pleura) with at least one of the following features: • Invasion of the endothoracic fascia. • Extension into the mediastinal fat. • Solitary, completely resectable focus invading soft tissues of the chest wall. • Non-transmural involvement of the pericardium
T4	Tumour involving all the ipsilateral pleural surfaces with at least one of the following features: • Diffuse or multifocal invasion of soft tissues of the chest wall. • Any rib involvement. • Invasion of the peritoneum through the diaphragm. • Invasion of any mediastinal organ. • Direct extension to the contralateral pleura. • Invasion of the spine or brachial plexus. • Transmural invasion of the pericardium (with or without pericardial effusion) or myocardium invasion
N	
Nx	Regional lymph nodes not assessable
N0	No regional lymph node metastases
N1	Metastases in the ipsilateral bronchopulmonary, hilar, or mediastinal lymph nodes (including the internal mammary, peridiaphragmatic, pericardial fat pad, or intercostal lymph nodes)
N2	Metastases in the contralateral bronchopulmonary, hilar, or mediastinal lymph nodes or ipsilateral or contralateral supraclavicular lymph nodes
M	
Mx	Presence of distant metastases not assessable
M0	No evidence of distant metastases
M1	Evidence of distant metastases

Table 3. TNM staging

Stage		T	N	M
I	a	T1	N0	M0
	b	T2	N0	M0
		T3	N0	M0
II		T1	N1	M0
		T2	N1	M0
III	a	T3	N1	M0
	b	T1	N2	M0
		T2	N2	M0
		T3	N0	M0
IV		T4	Any	Any
		Any	Any	M1

The most used staging method is that proposed by the International Mesothelioma Interest Group. The parameters considered are tumour extension (T), lymph node involvement (N) and metastatic dissemination (M) (Table 2). Combining these different parameters makes it possible to assign a stage to each patient (Table 3). Stage I indicates a neoplasm confined exclusively to the pleura in the absence of lymph node or metastatic localisation, while stage IV represents advanced inoperable disease. Staging is based on the patient's clinical picture, which is carried out employing instrumental investigations (especially CT and, where available, PET or PET/CT) and surgical procedures such as mediastinoscopy and video-thoracoscopy (VATS). Surgery can assess lymph node involvement (especially of N2 stations). Endoscopic techniques such as endobronchial ultrasound (EBUS) or oesophageal ultrasound (EUS) allow mediastinal involvement to be investigated.

Treatment

The treatment of MPM is a controversial issue due to the existence of different guidelines. It is generally resistant to traditional anticancer treatments (surgery, chemotherapy, and radiotherapy), but some progress has been made to introduce multimodality treatment. Survival gains, however, remain very modest.

Pleuropneumonectomy is a highly demolition surgical procedure, consisting of the en bloc removal of the pleura with the underlying lung, the pericardium, the loco-regional lymph nodes and the ipsilateral hemidiaphragm. It aims to eliminate any visible tumour focus). It is a procedure that is used less and less frequently because of the high perioperative risk and the mortality and morbidity rate. This option is considered in the early stages of the disease, when the neoplasm is shown to be confined to a hemithorax, in the absence of pericardial, diaphragmatic, and mediastinal invasion. The major postoperative complications are broncho-pleural fistula, haemothorax, empyema, pulmonary embolism, arrhythmias, respiratory failure, and heart failure.

Partial pleurectomy/decortication, on the other hand, consists of the partial or subtotal removal of the parietal and visceral pleura. This surgical technique, which is undoubtedly less demolitive than pleuropneumonectomy, guarantees a significant cytoreduction of the neoplasm, a gain in survival and responsiveness to adjuvant treatments. The main disadvantage is the absence of oncological radicality, which adds to the possibility of distant disease recurrence.

The approach, however, remains very invasive, as it is challenging to remove the visceral pleura from the lung. It is not uncommon to find significant air and/or blood leaks, which inevitably complicate the postoperative course. Therefore, in routine clinical practice, this is a palliative procedure that consists of partial or subtotal removal of flaps of parietal pleura and careful removal of the more exuberant portions of the visceral pleura (debulking). This procedure, if performed correctly, has the objective of a good re-expansion of the lung parenchyma.

Radiotherapy is widely used as a treatment for MPM, both for radical and palliative and analgesic purposes. Although MPM is erroneously considered a radioresistant neoplasm, the main problem is to deliver doses that have a radical effect (greater than 50 Gy) due to the extension of the surface to be irradiated and the presence, within the target volume, of anatomical structures with limited levels of radiation tolerance (lung parenchyma, spinal cord, heart). When performed for palliation purposes, radiotherapy effectively reduces or eliminates common symptoms such as chest pain, dyspnoea, dysphagia, and superior vena cava syndrome. However, its results in improving prognosis are poor, and the gain in months of survival is minimal.

While early-stage (stage I) is reserved for loco-regional surgical and/or radiotherapy approaches, later stages of MPM are treated with chemotherapy, which is especially effective in treating epithelioid and biphasic histotypes. Combined treatments generally produce better results than monotherapy, most notably the protocol of cisplatin and pemetrexed (or raltitrexed).

Chemical pleurodesis (pleural talcage) is reserved for patients with advanced diseases to ensure malignant pleural effusions. It consists of the thoracoscopic installation of sterile powder into the pleural cavity. Talc, a highly inflammatory substance, induces the formation of tenacious adhesions between the visceral and parietal pleura, obliterating the pleural cavity and preventing the effusion from forming again. After the complete evacuation of the effusion, it is necessary to check whether the lung can fully re-expand to ensure adhesion between the two pleural leaflets. If this is not the case, talcage should be avoided, as it would not be effective. A permanent pleural drain can be placed for purely palliative purposes, or a pleuroperitoneal or pleuropericardial window can be made.

REFERENCES

Baas P, Fennell D, Kerr K M, et al. Malignant pleural mesothelioma: ESMO Clinical Practice Guidelines for diagnosis, treatment and follow-up. *Ann. Oncol.* 2015 Sep; 26 Suppl 5:v31-9. doi: 10.1093/annonc/ mdv199.

Bueno R, Opitz I; IASLC Mesothelioma Taskforce. Surgery in Malignant Pleural Mesothelioma. *J. Thorac. Oncol.* 2018;13(11):1638-1654. doi: 10.1016/j.jtho.2018.08.001.

Kostron A, Friess M, Inci I, et al. Propensity matched comparison of extrapleural pneumonectomy and pleurectomy/decortication for mesothelioma patients. *Interact. Cardiovasc. Thorac. Surg.* 2017;24(5): 740-746. doi: 10.1093/icvts/ivw422.

Pelosi G, Papotti M, Righi L, et al. Pathologic Grading of Malignant Pleural Mesothelioma: An Evidence-Based Proposal. *J. Thorac. Oncol.* 2018; 13(11):1750-1761. doi: 10.1016/j.jtho.2018.07.002.

Scherpereel A, Opitz I, Berghmans T, et al. ERS/ESTS/EACTS/ESTRO guidelines for the management of malignant pleural mesothelioma. *Eur. Respir. J.* 2020;55(6):1900953. doi: 10.1183/13993003.00953-2019.

Travis W D, Brambilla E, Burke A P, et al. *WHO Classification of Tumours of the Lung, Pleura, Thymus and Heart*. 4th edition 2015, WHO Press.

van Zandwijk N, Clarke C, Henderson D, et al. Guidelines for the diagnosis and treatment of malignant pleural mesothelioma. *J. Thorac. Dis.* 2013; 5(6):E254-307. doi: 10.3978/j.issn.2072-1439.2013.11.28.

Wright C, Verma V, Barsky A R, et al. Quantitation and predictors of short-term mortality following extrapleural pneumonectomy, pleurectomy/ decortication, and nonoperative management for malignant pleural mesothelioma. *J. Thorac. Dis.* 2020;12(11):6476-6493. doi: 10.21037/

INDEX

A

adenocarcinoma, 56, 66, 107, 108, 120, 121, 125, 128, 129, 131, 134, 152
adhesion, 67, 80, 121, 124, 157
angiogenesis, 7, 13, 70, 80, 90, 92, 95, 107, 126
antibody, 11, 17, 18, 22, 27, 69, 70, 83, 84, 121
anti-CTLA4, 17, 18
antigen, 8, 11, 15, 26, 31, 68, 75, 82, 100, 120
antigen-presenting cells (APCs), 26
anti-PD-1, 17, 24
antitumor, 6, 11, 17, 30, 61, 66, 67, 69, 70, 71, 80, 111
antitumor agent, 61
asbestos, vii, ix, x, 3, 4, 5, 14, 15, 37, 42, 48, 52, 53, 54, 55, 56, 58, 59, 73, 74, 75, 76, 103, 116, 117, 125, 126, 127, 130, 131, 132, 133, 135, 137, 145, 146, 149
avelumab, 21, 41

B

benefits, 17, 21, 61, 110
benign, x, 56, 77, 119, 125, 141, 142, 143
biological fluids, 128
biomarkers, viii, 2, 13, 77, 107, 116, 118, 119, 127, 128, 129, 132, 133, 136
biopsy, 57, 59, 119, 144, 150
blood, 9, 71, 77, 90, 92, 94, 95, 104, 106, 107, 118, 136, 156
blood transfusion, 71
breast cancer, 105, 147

C

cancer, vii, ix, x, 3, 4, 5, 6, 7, 12, 14, 17, 26, 31, 34, 54, 58, 60, 63, 67, 68, 70, 71, 72, 74, 75, 79, 81, 82, 83, 84, 87, 88, 89, 90, 92, 93, 94, 95, 96, 101, 102, 103, 105, 106, 109, 110, 116, 118, 119, 124, 125, 127, 128, 129, 131, 142, 146
cancer cells, 5, 7, 26, 63, 68, 72, 118, 128
cancer progression, 90, 95
cancer therapy, 119

cancerous cells, ix, 54, 72, 88, 92, 101, 102
carcinogen, 54, 146
carcinogenesis, ix, 4, 15, 54, 88
carcinogenicity, 122
carcinoma, 83, 120, 121, 124
CCR, 35, 37, 41, 44, 48, 103, 106, 134
CD8+, 4, 6, 8, 9, 10, 11, 12, 15, 27, 31, 81
cellular therapy, 31
chemotherapy, viii, ix, 1, 2, 3, 5, 6, 17, 19, 22, 23, 24, 25, 27, 29, 32, 34, 52, 57, 59, 60, 61, 62, 65, 66, 67, 71, 73, 78, 84, 89, 94, 97, 101, 105, 106, 111, 156, 157
chromosomal abnormalities, 14
chromosome, 56, 123, 125
chronic illness, 93
chronic inflammation, 3, 4, 90, 93, 98
clinical application, 106
clinical presentation, 57
clinical trials, x, 8, 17, 21, 24, 27, 29, 31, 34, 66, 70, 71, 72, 79, 125, 142
colorectal cancer, 107, 109
combination of ICIs, 21
combination therapy, 33
complications, 62, 89, 100, 101, 110, 143, 156
controversial, 59, 88, 100, 155
correlation, 8, 27, 73, 116, 125
CSF, 5, 6, 15, 16, 28, 29, 36, 39, 45
cytokines, 4, 5, 15, 68, 83, 91, 93, 100, 101

D

DC therapy, 32
decortication, ix, 59, 60, 64, 78, 87, 88, 89, 95, 100, 101, 102, 111, 156, 158
dendritic cell, 6, 15, 100, 110
diaphragm, 56, 60, 64, 144, 150, 154
differential diagnosis, 120, 121, 122, 123, 125, 126, 133, 152
disease progression, 19, 22, 94

diseases, 56, 93, 119, 120, 122, 125, 126, 128, 136, 148, 157
DNA, 4, 15, 54, 65, 74, 75, 122, 123, 127, 146
DNA damage, 4, 15, 146
DNA repair, 122, 123
drainage, x, 63, 65, 113, 142, 150
drugs, 9, 34, 119, 125
durvalumab, 21, 22, 25, 37

E

effusion, 77, 136, 147, 157
epidermal growth factor, 7
European Medicines Agency, 23
evidence, ix, 16, 17, 23, 59, 63, 65, 70, 88, 95, 137, 154
exposure, vii, viii, x, 3, 4, 14, 51, 52, 53, 54, 56, 58, 59, 61, 73, 116, 130, 135, 145, 146, 149

F

fever, 54, 94, 99, 147
fibers, 3, 4, 14, 15, 54, 73, 103
fluid, 8, 54, 118, 126, 151
functional analysis, 9

G

gene expression, 11, 12, 114, 127, 128
gene therapy, 68
gene transfer, 84
genes, 11, 13, 65, 122, 127, 128, 146
granulocytic myeloid-derived suppressor cells (Gr-MDSCs), 7, 8, 42
growth, viii, 1, 4, 5, 7, 64, 65, 66, 67, 68, 70, 81, 90, 92, 95, 125, 126, 128
guidelines, 58, 89, 120, 155, 158

Index

H

hemoglobin, 90, 93, 97
hepatocyte growth factor, 7
heterogeneity, 10, 13, 30, 34, 93
histological examination, 144
histology, xi, 10, 11, 20, 23, 66, 72, 93, 99, 142, 143
histone deacetylase, 65, 79
history, vii, viii, 51, 52, 54, 57, 58, 59, 149
human, 8, 14, 22, 27, 29, 55, 70, 71, 74, 83, 104, 105, 110, 124
human body, 55
human neutrophils, 104
humoral immunity, 17

I

immune check-point inhibitors, viii, 2, 3, 16, 24
immune function, 110
immune modulation, 10, 100
immune reaction, 16
immune response, vii, ix, 8, 12, 13, 17, 26, 31, 68, 83, 88, 89, 90, 92, 100, 109, 125, 128
immune system, viii, ix, 2, 3, 5, 13, 16, 68, 69, 71, 72, 88, 89, 100, 101, 102, 127
immunity, ix, 16, 28, 84, 88, 90, 96, 102, 108
immunohistochemistry, 11, 59, 120, 123, 131, 151, 152
immunosuppression, 30, 69, 70, 100
immunotherapy, v, vii, viii, ix, 1, 2, 3, 5, 6, 10, 12, 13, 16, 26, 27, 28, 29, 30, 31, 32, 33, 34, 36, 38, 39, 40, 41, 42, 44, 46, 49, 60, 68, 69, 70, 81, 82, 88, 102, 111, 127
incidence, viii, x, 2, 34, 51, 52, 53, 55, 64, 73, 74, 116, 119, 145
inflammation, ix, 3, 4, 14, 53, 54, 82, 88, 89, 90, 91, 94, 95, 96, 97, 98, 99, 101, 103, 104, 109, 126, 145
inhibition, 6, 31, 67, 93, 122
inhibitor, 18, 21, 66, 67, 70, 80, 81, 146
ionizing radiation, viii, 51, 53, 55
ipilimumab, viii, 2, 3, 12, 19, 20, 21, 22, 23, 25, 29, 35, 39, 47, 48
ipsilateral, 60, 144, 149, 154, 156

L

lung cancer, viii, 17, 51, 53, 56, 60, 66, 74, 77, 80, 81, 83, 96, 97, 101, 103, 107, 108, 111
lymph node, 56, 58, 150, 154, 155, 156
lymphocytes, ix, 4, 9, 10, 68, 88, 92, 104, 105
lymphoma, 54, 65, 74, 143, 147

M

malignant mesothelioma, v, vii, viii, ix, x, 2, 3, 4, 5, 10, 14, 16, 17, 18, 19, 29, 32, 35, 36, 39, 40, 41, 42, 43, 46, 47, 51, 52, 53, 58, 59, 73, 74, 75, 76, 77, 78, 79, 80, 81, 84, 85, 99, 104, 106, 107, 116, 117, 120, 122, 123, 130, 131, 132, 133, 135, 138, 151
malignant pleural mesothelioma, v, vii, viii, ix, x, 1, 2, 3, 5, 6, 7, 8, 9, 10, 11, 12, 13, 15, 19, 20, 21, 22, 23, 24, 25, 27, 28, 29, 30, 31, 33, 35, 36, 37, 38, 39, 40, 41, 42, 43, 44, 45, 46, 47, 48, 51, 53, 56, 57, 59, 61, 72, 74, 75, 76, 77, 78, 79, 80, 81, 82, 83, 84, 85, 87, 88, 91, 93, 94, 95, 98, 99, 101, 102, 103, 104, 106, 107, 108, 109, 111, 130, 131, 132, 133, 134, 137, 138, 142, 143, 144, 157, 158
melanoma, 17, 31, 74, 146
membranes, x, 26, 141, 142

mesothelial, viii, 3, 4, 14, 15, 51, 54, 69, 116, 120, 124, 127, 135, 145, 151
metastasis, 56, 63, 64, 90, 95, 105, 110
monoclonal antibody, 10, 17, 66, 69, 70, 71, 82, 120, 121, 125, 135
monocytic myeloid-derived suppressor cells (Mo-MDSCs), 8
mortality, 60, 62, 72, 76, 88, 93, 94, 96, 116, 156, 158

N

neoplasm, viii, x, 1, 5, 51, 52, 142, 144, 145, 150, 155, 156
nivolumab, viii, 2, 3, 12, 19, 20, 21, 22, 23, 24, 25, 29, 35, 37, 39, 40, 44, 46, 47, 48
Nivolumab, 3, 12, 19, 20, 21, 22, 23, 24, 25, 29, 35, 37, 39, 40, 44, 46, 47, 48
nodal involvement, 56

O

objective response rate, 16
organs, vii, 54, 58, 64, 65
ovarian cancer, 31, 62, 82, 134

P

pain, 56, 63, 65, 72, 97, 143, 147, 148, 153, 157
palliative, 59, 61, 78, 156, 157
pancreatic cancer, 82, 95
paraneoplastic syndrome, 147
parenchyma, 145, 147, 154, 156, 157
pathogenesis, viii, 2, 14, 100, 105
pembrolizumab, 13, 18, 19, 24, 33, 35, 39, 43, 45
pericardium, viii, x, 51, 52, 53, 58, 60, 116, 124, 142, 144, 154, 156
peripheral blood, 31, 81, 91, 94, 104

peritoneal cavity, 57, 62
peritoneum, viii, x, 51, 52, 53, 58, 116, 124, 142, 144, 147, 154
phenotype, 5, 6, 10, 11, 12, 15, 96, 128, 146
placebo, 3, 18, 19, 66, 71, 79, 80
plasma cells, 11
platelet count, 91, 95
platelets, ix, 88, 90, 91, 95, 104, 147
platinum, viii, 1, 3, 21, 22, 23, 33, 61, 62, 67, 107
pleura, viii, x, 51, 52, 56, 58, 60, 116, 124, 131, 135, 141, 142, 143, 144, 149, 151, 154, 155, 156, 157
pleural cavity, 3, 59, 144, 157
pleural effusion, x, 31, 56, 57, 59, 70, 83, 123, 126, 142, 144, 147, 149, 151, 157
pneumonectomy, ix, 60, 64, 76, 77, 78, 79, 87, 88, 89, 94, 95, 97, 100, 101, 102, 103, 106, 111, 158
population, 18, 68, 92, 94, 95, 122, 135
positron emission tomography, 77, 99, 150
prognosis, vii, 5, 7, 10, 11, 12, 13, 34, 56, 72, 89, 91, 92, 93, 94, 95, 96, 97, 98, 99, 102, 103, 106, 109, 111, 116, 119, 126, 127, 129, 153, 157
pro-inflammatory, 54, 91, 92, 100, 102
proliferation, 8, 10, 15, 67, 100, 123, 125, 128, 146
proteins, 9, 65, 71, 76, 80, 100, 118, 124, 146
pulmonary embolism, 156
pulmonary function test, 57

R

radiation, ix, 52, 54, 55, 60, 63, 74, 76, 78, 79, 157
radiation therapy, 60, 63, 76
radiotherapy, ix, 33, 59, 88, 147, 156, 157
recruiting, 7, 15, 24, 25, 29, 67, 71

recurrence, 59, 64, 65, 72, 89, 101, 110, 143, 144, 156
resection, ix, x, 57, 60, 61, 78, 87, 89, 101, 103, 108, 142, 144
response, 4, 8, 11, 13, 16, 18, 21, 24, 25, 27, 32, 61, 62, 65, 67, 69, 89, 90, 97, 98, 100, 101, 105, 109, 110, 119, 125, 135, 145
risk, vii, viii, x, 4, 51, 53, 54, 55, 56, 59, 64, 74, 94, 97, 98, 99, 101, 102, 116, 119, 123, 125, 130, 144, 145, 146, 156

S

safety, 21, 22, 24, 25, 27, 31, 58, 66, 83, 88
sensitivity, 120, 124, 126, 129, 149
serum, 57, 91, 98, 99, 102, 123, 126, 134, 151
solid tumors, 13, 16, 26, 29, 31, 69, 80, 103
somatic mutations, 55, 74, 122, 131
superior vena cava syndrome, 147, 157
suppression, 5, 9, 68, 83, 84, 89, 127
surgical intervention, 96
surgical resection, 25, 57, 94, 101
surgical technique, x, 78, 142, 156
symptoms, x, 2, 56, 57, 94, 99, 109, 118, 142, 148, 149, 153

T

testis, viii, 51, 52, 58, 59, 75, 116
therapeutic approaches, 129, 130
therapeutic targets, 65, 118, 119
therapy, x, 13, 19, 22, 27, 31, 60, 63, 64, 65, 68, 79, 83, 106, 116, 124, 127, 138, 142
thoracoscopy, 59, 63, 101, 111, 155
thoracotomy, 101, 111, 144
tissue, vii, 5, 7, 8, 9, 10, 12, 14, 26, 56, 64, 65, 68, 75, 92, 96, 97, 100, 118, 151, 152
toxicity, 16, 19, 21, 31, 60, 62, 64, 65, 70

transformation, 3, 15, 127, 146
transforming growth factor, 7, 70
treatment, vii, viii, ix, x, 1, 2, 3, 10, 16, 17, 18, 20, 21, 22, 24, 26, 27, 31, 34, 57, 59, 60, 61, 62, 63, 65, 68, 74, 78, 83, 88, 89, 97, 98, 102, 105, 112, 116, 119, 123, 125, 127, 129, 130, 135, 141, 142, 144, 153, 155, 156, 157, 158
tremelimumab, 17, 18, 21, 36, 37, 43, 71, 84
trial, viii, 2, 3, 17, 18, 21, 22, 23, 27, 31, 60, 63, 65, 66, 68, 69, 70, 71, 78, 79, 80, 82, 83, 84, 88, 93, 105, 110
tumor cells, 6, 8, 13, 16, 26, 31, 69, 70, 71, 90, 98
tumor development, 65, 68, 92
tumor growth, 10, 30, 65, 91
tumor invasion, 69
tumor microenvironment, 4, 8, 15, 30, 43, 90, 91
tumor mutational burden, 13
tumor necrosis factor, 5
tumor necrosis factor-alpha, 5
tumor progression, 4, 6, 7, 9, 10, 91, 92, 95, 138

V

vaccines, 16, 26, 27, 30, 33, 37, 39, 40, 46
vascular endothelial growth factor receptor 2, 13
viral infection, 54, 55
viruses, ix, 52, 68, 71, 72

W

weight loss, 56, 72, 94, 97, 147
wound healing, 96, 108
wound infection, 72

CANCER ETIOLOGY, DIAGNOSIS AND TREATMENTS

MESOTHELIOMA

RISK FACTORS, TREATMENT AND PROGNOSIS

CANCER ETIOLOGY, DIAGNOSIS AND TREATMENTS

Additional books and e-books in this series can be found on Nova's website under the Series tab.